Nursing is a complex business,

requiring a high degree of context-specific coordination and communication among people with different skills and backgrounds. It seems that synergies among caregivers must be softly and flexibly assembled and disassembled to meet unpredictable situations, ready to become something else in an instant. New competencies and collaborations have to be seamlessly assimilated to improve the care giving process without disrupting it.

In the face of complexity and escalating costs, what can be done to ensure the bottom line that the patient gets well? What changes in education are needed to prepare nurses for the problems they face today and tomorrow? What new knowledge and understanding will nurses need at their fingertips?

The present volume brings together experts from multiple disciplines to address these and other problems in light of an emerging science of complex systems. Primary themes include self-organization as a source of pattern formation and change, interactivity and the notion of complex adaptive systems. The editors, who are also leaders and authors, are to be congratulated in being the first to bring insights and ideas from complexity theory to the field of nursing and to present them in such a coherent and highly accessible form. This volume should appeal to all concerned with nursing and the nursing environment, including patients and their families. The many rich examples cited throughout suggest a two-way learning process: The issues surrounding nursing and the healthcare system may also usefully inform and even shape the agenda of Complexity Science.

J. A. Scott Kelso, PhD founded the Center for Complex Systems and Brain Sciences at Florida Atlantic University (FAU). He holds the Creech Chair in Science at FAU and the Pierre de Fermat Chair of Excellence at the University of Toulouse and is the author of *Dynamic Patterns: the Self-Organization of Brain and Behavior* and (with David Engstrøm) *The Complementary Nature*, both published by The MIT Press.

On the Edge:
Nursing in the Age of Complexity

Claire Lindberg
Sue Nash
Curt Lindberg

PlexusPress
Bordentown, New Jersey

PlexusPress
www.PlexusInstitute.org

Cover and design by David Hutchens, Iconoclast Communications

ISBN: 1438246765

Contents

Dedication vii
Foreword ix
Preface. xiii

1. The Challenge of Change 1
   by Marjorie S. Wiggins

2. Nurses Take Note: A Primer on Complexity Science. 23
   by Curt Lindberg & Claire Lindberg

3. Complexity and Nursing Theory:
   A Seismic Shift. 49
   by Mary L. Gambino

4. Taking Complexity Science Seriously:
   New Research, New Methods 73
   by Ruth A. Anderson & Reuben R. McDaniel, Jr.

5. A Physicist Looks at Physiology 97
   by Bruce J. West

6. Beyond the Bedside: Nursing as Policy Making 125
   by Brenda Zimmerman & San Ng

7. A Möbius Band:
Paradoxes of Accountability for Nurse Managers. 159
    by Deborah Tregunno & Brenda Zimmerman

8. Walking with Families 185
    by Sue Nash

9. Thoughts on Thinking with Complexity in Mind 211
    by Daniel Pesut

10. The Challenge of Change: Inspiring Leadership. 239
    by James W. Begun & Kenneth R. White

Resource Guide and Glossary
of Nonlinear/Complex System Terms. 263
    by Jeffrey Goldstein

        Afterword. 295
        Acknowledgements. 299
        Index 301

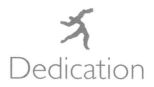

Dedication

This book is dedicated to the memory of Dr. Colleen P. Kosiak (1955 – 2006), a nurse educator, practitioner, and leader at the University of Kansas whose passion and commitment to nursing and advanced practice were filled with appreciation for the complexities of relationships among patients and healthcare professionals and who persisted in nurturing them. She was a true aficionado of Complexity Science and its promise to enlighten clinical, educational and organizational practices. May this book inspire others in their quest for deep knowledge, consistent with Dr. Kosiak's practices.

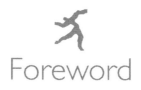

Foreword

In a dynamic environment, one must understand the potential of one. A small change can make a big difference. When nurses believe healthcare is unchangeable, when they see themselves as inconsequential parts of an unyielding system, they lose their ability to seize the moment. They think they have no ability to create change. Nothing could be further from the truth. Nurses must understand their critical role as healthcare leaders. The vast size and diversity of the nursing profession positions it for extraordinary influence on policy and practice in the twenty-first century. Indeed, the Institute of Medicine's reports, *To Err is Human* and *Crossing the Quality Chasm*, emphasize that care-giving at the individual level is a pivotal answer to solving the healthcare crisis. Human beings in need seek nurses to provide the human caring required to maintain optimum health. Nurses provide this service through a complex set of interactions that draw upon their skills in understanding human physiology, interpersonal psychology, sociological norms, financial constraints, cultural competency, pharmacology, and leadership.

What binds nurses together is the desire to give care to individuals in need using a sophisticated understanding built upon academic learning, life experiences, and a basic desire to make a difference. Holistic *caring* for individuals, families, and communities is the core objective for nurses.

Our society has yet to fully value the nursing profession for its profound commitment to this objective. Recognizing this with an understanding of the pressing healthcare needs around the world, nurses must reclaim their roots in activism to ensure better health for all. The world needs nurses who can practice within the full scope and capability of their profession, and by doing so, improve our broken system. More than ever, nurses must be capable change agents with a broadening world-view that embraces Complexity Science. Nurses use their assessment, critical thinking, and communication skills to help individuals, families, and communities with difficult health issues. Working alongside others, nurses examine the diversity of variables impacting health decisions. While not understood as such, nurses assist others in sensemaking as they make critical health-related choices and then cope with the outcomes through self-organization and adaptation. As change agents in a risk-laden environment, nurses must learn to live with paradox and uncertainty, and appreciate that hope is possible when unpredictability reigns.

According to the Institute of Medicine, the future healthcare system should be safe, effective, patient-centered, timely, efficient, and equitable. Prior attempts to manage care were cost-driven with documented healthcare detriment. As a response to these failed initiatives, the American Nurses Association promoted research to identify nurse-sensitive indicators that reflect the value of nursing care to produce positive health outcomes. Simultaneously, healthcare leadership is focusing on the improvement of patient care quality and safety. All healthcare practitioners, including nurses, must expand their understanding of how quality and safety can be achieved within complex systems.

In a broken system, turbulence is a necessary element in the process for change. Nurses in every aspect of practice are encouraged in this book to unlearn the linear teachings of the mechanistic world-view and competently embrace Complexity Science. Nurse educators have a special responsibility to prepare the next generation to practice with the knowledge of dynamic systems.

I have worked in nursing for thirty years as a staff nurse, administrator, educator, and now a dean. In my early experiences as the first line manager of an emergency department serving the medically uninsured and underinsured, I witnessed compassionate physicians, nurses, and allied health professionals who became increasingly frustrated with their inability to give optimal care. Possessed of these experiences, I sought more knowledge to build a deeper and richer understanding of the healthcare system. Now, twenty years later, I have witnessed many trends in healthcare innovation, but none that has satisfied the basic mandate to provide human beings with equitable opportunities to maintain health.

My nursing education emphasized the value of a theoretical framework for nursing practice. I learned that through interactions with others that one co-creates reality. Yet over my career I continued to experience a conflict between my unitary world-view and the logical, linear processes that regulated the reality of my practice. I was looking for Complexity Science long before I discovered it. And now I hope that you too will immerse yourself in the reflections presented in this outstanding book to begin the journey of adaptation, emergence, and a new world-view.

Dr. Cynthia Hornberger
Dean and Professor
Washburn University
April 16, 2008

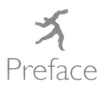

Preface

The science of complexity…helps us to see the world through a different lens, to make a fundamental shift in perception—from complexity as obstacle to complexity as opportunity.*

The roots of this book go back to the original White Paper on the Role of the Clinical Nurse Leader (American Association of Colleges of Nursing, 2004). One of us (Claire) was reviewing that document to develop a new graduate nursing curriculum and noticed the mention of "Complexity Theory" in the curriculum framework. Since another one of us (Curt) was already involved in educating healthcare professionals about Complexity Science, it seemed natural to team up and find ways to offer information on Complexity Science to nurse educators, nurse researchers, nursing leaders, and practicing nurses. Thus began the journey that produced this book.

Soon after, in April 2005, a conference sponsored by Plexus Institute and the Center for Complex Systems and Brain Sciences at Florida Atlantic University drew, among other participants, a number of nurses who were seeking insights into Complexity Science and their relevance to nursing

---

* Young, Eric. (2006). Foreword In. Westley, F., Zimmerman, B., & Quinn Patton, M., *Getting to Maybe: How the World is Changed*. Random House Canada.

practice. At this conference, we were blessed with a big open room with a smooth floor and chairs on wheels! We capitalized on those "wheely-chairs" to encourage mixing of conference participants and to move ideas around. One idea that repeatedly surfaced in the impromptu discussions: the pressing need for resources on Complexity Science and application of its principles in nursing. Many mentioned they would like to have a book that could be used by nurse educators as they sought to learn about and to integrate Complexity Science into their classes and curricula. Many also mentioned they would like to have a book for practicing nurses, nursing leaders, and students.

As the idea germinated and began to grow, we asked for volunteers. We had no idea who was going to be interested. The first person who popped up was our third editor, Sue Nash. Already a member of Plexus and an "early adopter" of Complexity Science in her classes at Augsburg College and in her family nursing practice, Sue was enthusiastic about "spreading the word" about Complexity Science in nursing. There, in the beautiful Florida sunshine, our editorial team was born.

Our next step was to develop the content of the book. In keeping with the principles of Complexity Science, we were looking for diversity, so we sought experts in complexity who were also interested in nursing as a profession. We reached out to some who we hoped would be interested in participating, but we also put out some "feelers" through the Plexus network. Authors responded with great ideas for topics and chapters. The authors chosen to participate have a deep interest in nursing and their own unique perspective on nursing, health, and healthcare. Thus, the book began to emerge. While we were working on building the contents of the book, nurses at conferences kept asking for references on Complexity Science, adding urgency to our task.

The result of three years of engagement, contribution, collaboration, and a little prodding, is the first comprehensive book on Complexity Science and Nursing. The chapters represent a survey of complexity concepts most relevant to nursing practice, research, and leadership. Chapter 1, by Marge Wiggins, sets the stage by providing an overview of the critical situation that exists in healthcare and nursing today. She describes threats to patient safety and the nursing workforce that have resulted from outdated leadership and healthcare delivery models and then proposes a new model to address these threats.

Lindberg & Lindberg's Chapter 2 provides an overview of some basic concepts of Complexity Science and relates them to examples from nursing. The stories and examples will resonate with nurses and nursing students who are faced with providing care to a sicker and more elderly population in an increasingly technological and multi-layered healthcare system. We suggest that readers who are "young" in their knowledge of Complexity Science start with these two chapters.

New theories and ideas are often met with resistance, particularly by those who are deeply invested in existing ones. Mary Gambino addresses this in Chapter 3. She explores the relationship of Complexity Science to nursing theory and practice. She takes the reader on a brief journey through the modern philosophy of science as it applies to nursing and argues that Complexity Science is more relevant to nursing practice today than some of nursing's historically important theories.

Ruth Anderson and Reuben McDaniel are the anchors in a leading network of researchers probing the implications of complexity for healthcare management and quality improvement. In Chapter 4 they present a comprehensive survey of the complexity-informed research methods they pioneered and their research on the association between management practices in nursing homes and patient outcomes.

It may take a few go-rounds for the reader to absorb the material in Chapter 5, but we believe if you stick with it, you will begin to reach new levels of understanding about the underlying dynamics of human health and illness. In this chapter, Bruce West demonstrates how medical and nursing interventions based on a traditional scientific and statistical thinking fall short in terms of addressing the physiologic actions of the body and the pathophysiologic dynamics of disease. It took each of us (Claire, Curt, & Sue) several exposures to West's ideas before we "got it" but when the "ah ha" arrived, we felt it was well worth the mental workout.

Chapter 6 by Brenda Zimmerman and San Ng takes us beyond the bedside, into the world of health policy. These authors explore healthcare policy from a traditional perspective and describe how Complexity Science opens up new views into the policy making process. These views are likely to stimulate greater participation by nurses in local, national, and global policy work. They illustrate how nurses' influence at the local level can affect health and healthcare nationally and internationally.

Deborah Tregunno and Brenda Zimmerman bring a Complexity Science perspective to nursing management in Chapter 7. They identify three fundamental paradoxes faced by today's nurse managers. Using the example of the widely different responses to the SARS epidemic in two Canadian cities, the authors demonstrate how the three paradoxes play out in practice.

All nursing is about families, according to Sue Nash, who examines how a Complexity Science perspective on family has the potential to enrich nurses' ability to promote health and healing in families. Chapter 8 takes us into nurse-family interactions through examples from Nash's own family nursing practice, those of her colleagues, and those of her RN-BSN students.

At the heart of nursing is how nurses think, reason, and make decisions. In Chapter 9, Dan Pesut presents a model that explains the iterative process through which nurses move from assessing data to diagnosis, choosing interventions and evaluating the results of nursing care. This chapter presents a new focus on more complex types of thinking that emphasizes pattern recognition. At the end of this chapter, we present some "food for thought" on how Pesut's model can evolve to further incorporate Complexity Science concepts. This chapter, along with the editor reflections, challenges the reader to examine clinical reasoning and judgment in depth, particularly in light of the increasing chronicity and complexity faced by patients and rapid technological advances in healthcare.

In Chapter 10, Jim Begun and Ken White look at nursing and the leadership potential of individual nurses, nursing organizations, and nursing as a profession. Assets existing in nursing are evaluated and critical leadership competencies are described. In a chapter that is both intriguing and empowering, Begun and White critically analyze nursing's ability to engage with three critical leadership competencies to further the profession's contributions in healthcare.

Chapter 11, the Resource Guide and Glossary by Jeffrey Goldstein, will help readers understand Complexity Science terms and concepts used in this book and will introduce more technical and advanced concepts. The chapter reference list contains a wealth of information on important resources as well.

We hope this book successfully conveys some basics on Complexity Science and its applications in nursing and healthcare to those who are beginning to explore the science. We also hope it will prove useful to those already on the journey or who are searching for new strategies to improve nursing and healthcare. We also expect that it will pique readers' interest in delving deeper into this exciting new science and learning more about how it can enhance their practice.

This book represents both an ending and a beginning. It is the end of a long, sometimes tedious, but often exciting journey from a need and an idea to the first comprehensive publication on Complexity Science and Nursing. It is also the beginning of what we hope will become a multitude of new journeys into the land of Complexity Science—yours and ours.

Claire Lindberg and Curt Lindberg

The Challenge of Change
by Marjorie S. Wiggins

Our lives are connected by a thousand invisible threads, and along these sympathetic fibers, our actions run as causes and return to us as results.[1]

The Period of Transformation

The development of the personal computer and easy access to the Internet has changed the way we live. Suddenly, with the ability to stroke a few keys, communication transitioned from face-to-face or phone conversations to text messages and e-mails. Our personal belongings now include handheld technology that connects us to friends across continents and oceans. The new technology has changed many of the simple daily activities in our lives. Shopping for groceries and buying clothes can be done in the living room on the computer. Information, including the latest from medicine, is readily available electronically. It is now possible for patients to have more current information about their medical condition than their doctors do. Rapid access to information has also contributed to advances in medical science and research, providing us with information that enables us to treat illnesses that were previously a mystery.

New technologies have improved our lives, made the world a much smaller place, and dramatically transformed the way we live and work. Medical technology has advanced as well. For example, the introduction of robotics in surgery allows surgeons to operate on patients without being in the same room or even the same country. The fine instrumentation used by robots combined with high-definition screens that magnify the surgical site have improved surgical precision, reducing nerve damage and bleeding.

Advances in information and technology have changed the way people work. Even though the healthcare industry relies on an abundance of technology, little has changed in the way direct care is delivered.

The world of the twenty-first century continues to change at a rate so rapid it is beyond comprehension. The foundation of the former industrialized economy has shifted from natural resources to intellectual assets, and with the shift has come a level of complexity that challenges us and provides increased opportunities for innovation and creativity.

Responding to Environmental Change

In many cases, advances in information and technology have changed the way people work. However, even though the healthcare industry relies on an abundance of technology, little has changed in the way direct care is delivered. Nursing, in particular, has struggled to rethink the way work is done and has floundered in its attempt to develop new models of care to organize that work.

A closer examination of the obstacles that have prevented progress in nursing is warranted. Nurses are at the sharp end of care. Within the hospital and in many other healthcare settings, nurses provide the most direct care to and have more contact with the patient than other healthcare providers. They are the professionals who monitor the patient's responses to treatments and therapies. It is the nurse who ensures coordination and effectiveness of patient care. Comprising the largest number of healthcare professionals in the United States, nurses have the greatest potential for improving individual patient outcomes as well as the overall safety and effectiveness of the healthcare industry. Because of their role as patient advocates, nurses are trusted by patients and their families. Nursing has the potential to be the strong voice for needed change in the healthcare arena.

Past is Prologue

Modern healthcare systems evolved during the industrial age of the late eighteenth and early nineteenth centuries. This era has significantly influenced the delivery of healthcare as we know it today. Industrial models of work were built on linear processes, with the classic example being the assembly line. In addition, the model for organizations was hierarchical, characterized by well-defined reporting and authority structures. The predominant model for healthcare delivery today exhibits similar linear processes and structures of hierarchy, authority, and control. Nursing, medicine, and other healthcare disciplines also have their origins in this era and display similar management structures, lines of authority, and unique practices and traditions. The educational institutions that developed during the industrial era supported discipline-specific learning and helped keep disciplines separate and distinct. Much of this educational legacy persists today.

For similar reasons, institutions that housed healthcare developed organizational structures, chains of command, defined policies, and roles.

Nursing:	Dietary:	Pharmacy:	Social work:	Pathology:	Radiology:	Physical therapy:
Processes, procedures, competencies, medications, schedules, staffing, assessments, documentation, families	Processes, procedures, calorie counts, nutrition assessment, special diets	Drugs, drugs, drugs, formulary, distribution, contraindications, inventory, adverse drug events	Family support groups, counseling centers, aedvisors, insurance & Medicaid application, financial management	Blood bank, laboratory, tests, diagnostics, phlebotomists, billing	X-ray, MRI, CAT scanners, films, techs, billing	Range of joint, activities, gym, exercise, rehab therapy, documentation, billing

Figure 1: Hospital organization showing departments as "silos"

These factors led to the establishment of separate and distinct departments responsible for defined tasks and roles. Figure 1 demonstrates the organization of most hospitals today. Existing departments are pictured as separate and distinct columns, depicting the uniqueness of the separate disciplines or departments as well as the boundaries that divide them. Organizational structures that function in relative isolation inside inflexible boundaries are sometimes referred to as "silos." The compartmentalization that supported specialization contributed to the development of such silos, which increased barriers to collaboration.

Despite compartmentalization, hospitals functioned relatively effectively for many years because of an excess of resources. Inefficiencies that existed were supported by elongating hospitals stays and adding more staff. The relatively slow pace of care allowed for communication and care delivery processes to proceed in a linear and uncomplicated fashion. The abundance of resources also allowed for development of new services and ancillary disciplines to support care. Patient care needs were also met by the development and growth of new provider roles, including advanced practice nurses and physician assistants. While each new role provided additional resources, the level of complexity involved in the provision of care increased dramatically. As more services and providers entered the scene, a need for care coordination arose and the case manager role was born. At the time, the healthcare reimbursement system rewarded care providers for doing more. An unforeseen consequence of the growth of specialized roles and services was rapid inflation in the cost of care.

Healthcare Costs Soar

Beginning in the 1970s, the expansion of healthcare technology and resources caused healthcare costs to skyrocket. The high cost of medical care and its exponential growth led to fear of unsustainable expense and a mandate for change. From 1980 to 1990, healthcare expenditures almost tripled, going from $253 billion in 1980 to $714 billion a decade later.[2] To halt the spiraling costs, dramatic changes were made in the way healthcare was reimbursed. The retrospective cost reimbursement schema that fueled the tremendous growth in services was replaced with the prospective payment system that provided incentives for decreased resource use. This shift in reimbursement policies proved to be a seminal event. As brakes were applied to spending and payment incentives were shifted, healthcare leaders realized that in order to financially survive, they would have to respond to the new rules of reimbursement.

Cost Cutting Impacts Care

One of the most significant initiatives undertaken to curtail costs was to decrease the length of time allotted for provision of patient care services inside and outside acute care settings. For example, in hospitals, the ten- to fourteen-day lengths of stay typical in the 1970s were halved. The need to decrease utilization of expensive hospital care also led to other changes. Dedicated units were created to provide pre-admission testing on an outpatient basis which eliminated one day in the hospital for surgical stays. New levels of intermediary care, sometimes called "step down units," were created so patients who no longer required critical care but were not ready for general unit care could be treated in a safe and cost-effective manner. Although this three-tier schema resulted in shorter lengths of stay, it also led to fragmented care which created new challenges. One of those challenges is commonly called "handoffs," which refers to the process of transferring patients between units or between groups of caregivers within a healthcare setting. Handoffs are now so frequent that the Joint Commission of Accreditation of Healthcare Organizations has required that processes be established to ensure complete and accurate communication between units and providers when patients are transferred. The role of the case manager was also affected. Case management shifted focus from its original purpose of patient management across the care continuum to utilization review and discharge planning. Utilization review and discharge planning are both processes that monitor the delivery of services to patients with an eye on providing care in the most cost-effective manner. Utilization review nurses monitor patients' conditions with the goal of providing a level of care that is safe and appropriate, but not excessive. An example is ensuring that patients are rapidly moved to a lower level of care (for instance, from a cardiac care unit to a telemetry or step-down unit) as soon as their condition permits. Likewise, discharge planning has as its goal the development of plans to move patients out of the hospital as quickly as possible to a nursing home, a rehabilitation setting, or their own home.

Throughout this period of massive change, nurses strove to provide the best possible care, but found themselves handicapped by the need to deliver care at an unprecedented pace. In 2001, Anita Tucker, then a doctoral candidate at the Harvard Business School, undertook a 200-hour observational study to examine nurses' work.[3] Results showed that nurses were working harder and faster than employees in other industries. The nurses in Tucker's study completed an average 160 separate tasks in a single eight-hour shift. Each task, on average, took two minutes and forty-eight seconds. Tucker noted that in order to keep up with the needs of patients, nurses worked at what she termed a "staccato pace." Tucker also observed the occurrence of errors (n=28) and problems (n=166) during the study period. Errors were defined as "executions of a task that is either unnecessary or incorrectly carried out."[4] Inherent in this definition is the idea that these errors could have been avoided if appropriate information had been communicated. Problems were defined as "a disruption in worker's ability to execute a prescribed task."[4] Errors and problems together were termed "failures." One hundred and ninety-four failures occurred during the study period.[4]

Tucker's work illustrates the obstacle course nurses navigate every day as they provide care. Many of these obstacles are related to failures within the system and not to actions by individual nurses. According to Begun and White, "nursing service delivery systems are interdependent with elements external to nursing: the profession of nursing is not well insulated from its environment."[5] In fact, nursing can never be isolated from the complexities and weaknesses of the healthcare environment as the nurse "lives where the patient lives" and is the link between all care providers and systems that support the patient. Traditionally, as nurses were faced with system failures within a fast-paced work environment, they compensated by applying band-aid solutions designed to meet immediate patient needs. An example is the nurse who, noticing that not enough linen is delivered each day to meet needs of the unit, repeatedly "borrows" linen from another unit. While these actions may show ingenuity and may solve an immediate problem, they do not address the root cause of the issue which lies within larger systems and processes.

Efforts and Errors

As the healthcare system tried to meet the dual challenges of expansion and expense reduction, cost-cutting measures took their toll. Healthcare providers began to exhibit signs of stress and burnout, and patient outcomes started to suffer. The U.S. healthcare system, once considered a worldwide gold standard, began to lose its ability to produce high-quality outcomes. In 2000, the Institute of Medicine publication *To Err is Human: Building a Safer Health Care System for the 21st Century* reported that 44,000 to 98,000 Americans were dying in U.S hospitals each year as the result of medical errors. This represents more deaths per year than from motor vehicle accidents (45,297), breast cancer (42,297), or AIDS (16,516).[6] The report stunned the healthcare community and caused concern in the American public. Many wondered how the most expensive healthcare system in the world could yield such poor results. Others wondered how so many fatal errors could occur despite years of emphasis on quality assurance, performance improvement, and continuing education. What factors prevented high-quality outcomes? A follow-up report published the next year, *Crossing the Quality Chasm: A New Healthcare System for the 21st Century*,[7] set forth a mandate for fundamental change in the healthcare system to ensure safe, effective, patient-centered care, delivered in a timely, efficient, and equitable manner. The report moved beyond assigning individual blame for medical errors and poor outcomes and recognized that problems related to safety and quality were systemic in nature and primarily related to outmoded systems of work.[7] These systemic problems arose at least in part because many of the systems in place were designed for the industrial era and did not meet current needs. The linear, mechanistic thinking of the industrial age cannot solve the problems of the information era—an age of complexity unlike any we have ever experienced.

Perhaps the biggest challenge faced by leaders in the healthcare field today is the need to move away from the mechanistic thinking of past eras when precision, standardization, control, and command were the hallmarks of efficient, well-managed organizations. As healthcare organizations have become more complex, departmental functions have become increasingly interdependent and department-specific efficiencies at times conflict with overall system efficiency. Rigid rules, standardized procedures, and policies can impede adaptation in an era of transformation and rapid change. Contrasting the characteristics of the healthcare system of the industrial age with the complex conditions existing today leads us to the realization that these old ways of thinking limit innovation and creativity. In healthcare and in nursing fundamental change is required. Tim Porter O'Grady, a futurist, recognized the need for change:

> The times indicate that our experience is not much different today from the time at the end of the 18th century when the trade guilds of Europe were becoming extinct....Holding on to old notions that no longer characterize the demands of the time will do nothing but exacerbate the conditions which facilitate the demise of nurses and nursing work.[8]

The mandate is clear. New thinking is necessary to solve the healthcare crisis. Nursing must take the lead. The level of change required will take

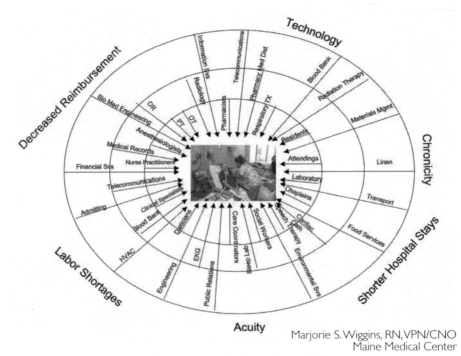

Marjorie S. Wiggins, RN, VPN/CNO
Maine Medical Center

Figure 2: The complexity of care delivery,

courage and a new mental model to help us achieve the transformation that is necessary.

Complexity Science in Healthcare

Hospitals and healthcare systems can be described as complex adaptive systems (CASs). Care of an acute care patient today literally involves hundreds of people. Figure 2 depicts many of the players who are involved directly or indirectly in delivering healthcare to one patient. What is important to understand in any CAS, and certainly in hospitals, is the interdependency among individual agents and groups. In a CAS, each agent acts on local knowledge and experience. If these agents are able to learn with and from each other, they will be better able to respond effectively to novel situations as they arise. The rigid rules, structures, and boundaries inherited from the past sometimes inhibit our ability to adapt in the dynamic, ever-changing environment of healthcare.

One busy summer evening, the emergency room of a large tertiary hospital was presented with a considerable number of acute patients. As patients were classified as needing admission, the admitting department was notified of the need to move the patients to regular hospital beds. The admitting department advised the ER staff that there were no beds available even though discharges had occurred and discharged patients had left for home. As precious time passed, more patients presented to the ER, including trauma victims and high acuity cardiac patients. At this point, the ER staff notified the supervisor that they were forced to go on diversion. Diversion means that ambulance drivers are notified to bypass the hospital ER and take patients to other hospitals. This is a very serious event as it essentially shuts down emergency services to the community. The supervisor, noting that patients had been discharged, yet there were no available in-patient beds, investigated the situation. It didn't take long for her to discover that all the housekeeping staff had gone on an extended dinner break together to celebrate a colleague's birthday. A one-hour interruption of the cleaning of beds brought the hospital admission process to a halt and caused a series of events to almost shut down service to the community.

One example of this interdependency is related to efforts to use hospital beds more efficiently. Occupancy rates have been tightened over the years in an effort to create efficiency by reducing vacancy rates. Where it was once common for hospitals to operate at seventy-five to eighty percent of their capacity, now these same institutions strive for ninety to ninety-five percent occupancy rates. This creates new challenges, including frequent lack of unoccupied beds. Bed availability is complicated by the unpredictability of demand. Emergency rooms may fill quickly with patients requiring inpatient care. To accommodate the flow of patients from the emergency room to inpatient units, bed turnover throughout the hospital must be efficient. This requires that beds vacated by discharges early in the day be readied quickly for admissions. For this system to function effectively, various elements involved in the process of discharging the patients, cleaning the beds and rooms, and transporting patients and supplies must communicate well and function smoothly together. Box 1 provides an example of how an unexpected event in such a system led to a backup of patients in the emergency room of one hospital with potentially serious consequences for individual patients and the community. The story illustrates the interdependence that exists in complex hospital systems today and is one of millions of examples of how individual agents are interwoven and interconnected in the care and service we provide to patients.

Revising Old Models of Care

When we look at the recent history of nursing, we see a pattern in the response to the changing landscape of healthcare: to work harder and faster to meet patient needs. There have been no significant changes in the way work is organized. The approach to care delivery has remained unchanged. The last major development in nursing care delivery design was the primary nursing model introduced in 1969 by Marie Manthey.[9] Primary nursing was based on the premise that one nurse assumed twenty-four hour accountability for the care of a patient or a group of patients. The model was comprised of four elements: 1) allocation of and acceptance of individual responsibility for decision making; 2) assignment of daily care by the case method; 3) direct person-to-person communication; and 4) operational responsibility for the quality of care administered to patients on a unit twenty-four hours a day, seven days a week by a single individual nurse.[9] Within this model, key aspects of care, including assessment, care planning, direct patient care, coordination of communication, measurement of progress, discharge planning, and patient and family education, would all be provided or directed by the primary nurse. Primary nursing was launched with the intention of decreasing the fragmentation of care. Today, many nurses, managers, and chief nurses have difficulty identifying the model that informs the delivery of care in their institution.

The underlying concept of a single nurse being responsible for a patient's care has succumbed to twelve-hour shift schedules, wherein full-time nurses work only three shifts per week. The phenomenon of moving patients among multiple units during a single hospital stay further complicates this picture. Given these factors, it is nearly impossible for a single nurse to assume responsibility for a patient's care during a hospital stay.

Patients and families are acutely aware of the high number of nurses and other professionals providing care in a hospital episode and notice the apparent lack of comprehensive knowledge of their case by any single hospital staff member. Many family members stay at the hospital daily to ensure all healthcare providers have accurate and complete information about their loved ones in the hopes of preventing the occurrence of critical medical errors.

Patient Care as Shared Responsibility

As discussed earlier, a healthcare delivery organization is a CAS composed of smaller CASs. For example, an intensive care unit (ICU) is a CAS within a hospital. Agents (people) in the ICU include patients, staff nurses, clinical nurse specialists, nurse practitioners, physicians, pharmacists, nurse managers, respiratory therapists, technicians, social workers, and secretaries. The ICU is only one of the many units, or CASs, that a patient may visit.

The complexity and the interdependency of agents who interact in a self-organizing manner make it impossible for any single agent to control the processes and outcomes of care for any patient. Care can no longer be considered the responsibility of one individual as in the Primary Nursing model but, of necessity, must be shared among many agents. Many times agents act on behalf of the patient without being aware of decisions and actions of other agents. For this very reason we must embrace a model of care that recognizes the existing diversity and the interconnectedness of agents in the healthcare system.

In an attempt to develop new models of care, nursing has limited its perspective to its own profession and has failed to recognize its place as a microsystem within a larger CAS. The ability for nursing to perform its critical role is highly dependant upon the work of others. For this reason, nursing must invite a variety of other players to develop a multidisciplinary approach to care. Only by embracing the diversity of all the agents involved in care delivery will nursing free itself from the isolation that has inhibited its ability to adapt and create new approaches to care. A new era requires new thinking. Patient care belongs to multiple disciplines and agents. Compartmentalized care limits and inhibits best outcomes. It is time to transition to a more flexible and collaborative care model. The expert model of individual disciplines needs to shift to one of partnership with all disciplines, the patient, and family.

Transition to a New Model of Care

Many fields, including nursing and healthcare management, are adopting the Complexity Science framework. By focusing on increasing connections, diversity, information flow, and interactions, nursing and other healthcare managers can foster creative self-organization or adaptation. Complexity Science builds on, and sometimes questions, the rich tradition of nursing that views patients and nursing care from a system perspective. A Complexity Science perspective suggests that relationships with and participation by a diverse group of agents and stakeholders may facilitate the creation of new and effective delivery systems.

Partnerships are Paramount

Nursing has long recognized the importance of relationships between nurses and patients, and patients and the environment or social system. Such systems thinking is evident in the work of several nurse theorists including Dorothy Johnson, Imogene King, Sister Calista Roy, and Margaret Newman.[10] Building on the strong foundation of systems thinking evident in nursing, it is possible to extend our understanding of this to care delivery in a complex environment. With Complexity Science as a framework, nursing is guided to engage in a high degree of collaboration with other stakeholders (agents) involved in patient care including, most important, those who have the most to gain (or lose) in the delivery of care: the patients and their families. All other agents must recognize the role played by patients and families in care and seek to form highly collaborative relationships or partnerships with them as well as with other professionals and caregivers. The word partnership, defined as "a relationship between individuals or groups that is characterized by mutual cooperation and responsibility as for the achievement of a specific goal,"[11] emphasizes the strength and intent of the relationship. Clearly, the goal for patient care is to achieve optimal outcomes for the patients we serve.

Building a care delivery model that recognizes multiple agents who are constantly interacting and changing in response to each other requires flexibility in planning and design. Sometimes, detailed planning and rigidly applied plans fail in complex, turbulent, political contexts where there are ambiguous objectives and divergent problems.[12] Certainly, vision needs to be provided as well as general goals and boundaries, but the abilities to explore, act on experience, and interact and respond to other agents are key in complex settings.

A new care delivery model in use at Maine Medical Center is the Partnership Care Delivery Model. This model was developed to address the recognized need for transformation to a more collaborative type of care that emphasizes patient safety and that puts patients and families at the center. Nursing plays a key role in this model although all disciplines and hospital departments participate. The role of the Clinical Nurse Leader® (CNL) is important in this model as is described below. In the case of the partnership model of care, the vision of safe patient- and family-centered care that values and respects the input of the patient and family creates the context of the model.[13] This model underscores the aim of patient centeredness set forth by the Institute of Medicine in its second report, which is to design safer healthcare systems.[7] The model is also grounded in the assumptions that care should be outcome-oriented as opposed to shift-specific, and it should be based on the best available scientific evidence. These specifications should guide disciplines in their search for care delivery innovations.

The time has passed for a care delivery model to rely simply on role descriptions, policies, or isolated disciplines such as nursing. Recognition that healthcare is a CAS requires us to acknowledge the existing complexity within the system as we try to move forward with fundamental changes for the way care is provided. Complexity Science promises new descriptive theoretical models for identifying organizational building blocks; understanding organizational behavior and structures and change; and fostering change at both the micro- and macrosystem levels.[12] Using a theory with these properties provides the opportunity for development of a model that is flexible and responsive and more likely to foster better outcomes for patients.

Partnership, the core concept of the new care delivery model, emphasizes the importance of relationships where members of the partnership are seeking mutual outcomes. The most significant partnership is that of the nurse with the patient and the family. Other partnerships include the nurse and the physician, and the nurse and professionals from other disciplines. The strength of the partnership is a key factor in achieving change at the clinical microsystem level.

Clinical microsystems are defined as small, functional frontline units where professionals provide most healthcare to people. Clinical microsystems are complex systems that have structure, some patterns of ordered relationship, and some processes. The processes are the means of connecting the patterns and structures to create the output and work.[14] Clinical microsystems are the essential building blocks of larger healthcare systems. The quality and value of care produced by a large healthcare system can be no better than the services generated by the small systems of which it is composed.[14] These microsystems are where patients, families, and care teams meet. It is in the clinical microsystem where we see the opportunity for change and improvement in the healthcare system. The immediate care teams of individual agents can work together to create change within their unique microsystem.

Within this model, a new role in nursing, the master's prepared Clinical Nurse Leader (CNL), has been created to work at the microsystem level to facilitate quality patient outcomes and performance improvement. The concept of the role was introduced in 2003 by the American Association of Colleges of Nursing in a document titled the *"White Paper on the Education and Role of the Clinical Nurse Leader."*[15] The role was developed in response to the error and patient safety issues noted in the IOM reports,[6;7] the growing nursing shortage, and the understanding that new competencies are required to ensure safe patient care. As the role has spread across the country, early outcomes demonstrate that education that stresses understanding the complex systems in which healthcare providers work, and skills to address issues at the microsystem level, are leading to improvements in care.

The CNL functions within a microsystem of care, often a nursing unit. The CNL role includes two primary functions: lateral integration of care and quality improvement. Lateral integration is accomplished by overseeing a case load of vulnerable, at-risk patients with complex care needs. In this role, the CNL is responsible for care coordination among all members of the multidisciplinary team. One method the CNL uses to ensure safe care is by making sure that each healthcare provider has information necessary to provide care no matter where the patient is within the hospital or along the continuum of care. The primary function of quality improvement projects is based on the CNL's advanced knowledge of risk analysis within the microsystem of care. Using this knowledge, the CNL identifies issues that affect quality of care or that may compromise patient safety, and works with all stakeholders to identify strategies to solve the root causes for these system failures. Identifying inefficiencies and errors at the microsystem level can have profound effects on the overall institution as well. For example, two CNLs at Maine Medical Center saved the hospital $1 million by working on two projects and bringing them to a positive conclusion. One involved reducing the number of days patients were on ventilators in the critical care unit. The result was an 18 percent decrease in ventilator days for all patients over a 14-month period. The second project involved eliminating the practice of re-transfusion of blood cells to patients who had undergone knee surgery. The latter project demonstrated that the re-transfusion did not result in an increase in patients' hematocrit levels. These transfusions were eliminated as a result of the CNL working with the orthopedic surgeons, other care providers, the patients, and families at the microsystem level. These two projects are described in more detail in the interview with Marjorie Wiggins that follows this chapter.

Future Directions

By being open to the new mental model Complexity Science provides, nursing can seize an opportunity to shed its current limitations and create a better healthcare system by working collaboratively with everyone involved in patient care. With new care delivery models and roles that recognize the complexity of today's environment and address delivery process failures, a new direction is possible for healthcare. The future holds great promise for patients and healthcare professionals when we use new thinking to address a new time.

Putting It All Into Practice

What follows is an interview with Marjorie Wiggins by Plexus Communications Director and Staff Writer, Prucia Buscell

Marjorie Wiggins's vision for nursing in the twenty-first century has emerged from devoted attention to detail, theoretical scholarship, empathy, and the infusion of lofty time-honored ideals into a high-tech environment.

After a fast-paced description of the myriad changes in healthcare, including new technology, new medicines, financial strains, and evolving work patterns, Ms. Wiggins observes that the only constants are patients and nurses. "We live where the patient lives. We are in the midst of all the systems that come together to take care of the patient," she says. "Because of where we live, our exposure, and our presence, nursing has the ability to make significant changes. Imagine if a population as big as nursing—that's 2.6 million nurses, the biggest healthcare population in the country—decided to do things differently, creating new roles, delivering new care models. "We can revolutionize the field. We are the safety net, and the sharp end of care. We see it all, hear it all, understand it all," she continues. "Nurses by nature are advocates for patients. If we can make changes at the micro level, across the country, we can carry a very strong voice into the future for patients and the improvement of patient care."

Ms. Wiggins has already put some of her beliefs into practice at Maine Medical Center, where she is vice president of nursing and chief nurse executive. Maine Medical Center is a 606-bed hospital in Portland, ME, with services in all medical specialties. In her capacity there, Ms. Wiggins was instrumental in developing the role of Clinical Nurse Leader (CNL) and a Partnership Model of Care Delivery at MMC. Both are designed to achieve the highest quality patient care and safety by having patients, families, and healthcare providers work closely together.

Ms. Wiggins served on an implementation task force for the American Association of Colleges of Nursing to foster the CNL role across the country, and she wanted it at home too. The CNL position, created in 2003, is the first new nursing role in four decades. CNLs have master's degree-level training in addition to their nursing degrees. They have an in-depth knowledge of medical decisions being made on behalf of the patients to whom they are assigned, and they understand the thinking and practice of different clinical disciplines. As a result, they can keep patients and families well informed. They're called "lateral integrators," Ms. Wiggins notes, because they keep track of the patient across a continuum of care, and across an entire hospital setting.

"We spent two years getting the environment ready to implement the CNL role," Ms. Wiggins says of her efforts at MMC. "We worked on making the care very patient centered, and developing partnerships with the patients, and we did a lot of explaining to others players—doctors, other nurses, management, the trustees. We did a lot of internal and external marketing." Ms. Wiggins has written articles about partnerships, which she describes as stronger than collaborations because they involve being invested in each other's goals to achieve mutual ends, and willingness to take risks together.

From a Complexity Science viewpoint, CNLs are local agents who work with interdisciplinary teams and who can create changes in healthcare microsystems. Ms. Wiggins learned about Complexity Science three years ago at a Plexus Institute conference at Hunterdon Medical Center, in Flemington, NJ, and the concepts immediately resonated with her. She began intensive reading and study, and started to see the world through a different lens. The new view gave her an intense appreciation for what happens in modern healthcare when literally hundreds of people may be involved in caring for one patient in a fast-paced, complex, and sometimes chaotic environment. She and her colleagues began developing numerous ways to get patients and families more involved in care.

When CNLs at MMC complete their academic training, they undergo immersion in the clinical setting, with seven weeks of appointments and interviews with people from departments throughout the hospital. They learn about the operations of dietary, housekeeping, infectious disease, and continuing care, among others, and as they learn broadly about the hospital's services, service providers learn what CNLs do. "We created stronger relationships among the members of the interdisciplinary team," Ms. Wiggins says.

Another learning initiative promoted patient involvement by having all providers sensitized to patient perspectives. In the MMC Partnership Care Delivery Model, all providers, doctors, nurses, pharmacists and caregivers discovered new insights through half hour interviews they conducted with patients or family members. "They learned what it's like to move from floor to floor and have different staff they don't know. They learned what it's like to not understand a diagnosis, or the medication," she says. "It was very beneficial. We think patients understand everything we tell them. They don't. We think they can navigate the healthcare system. They can't. We have different languages, different customs. It's like being in a different land."

To further patient care with patients in mind, MMC created advisory committees, one for adults and one for pediatrics, with patients or family members among the members. They advise on everything from how buildings should be built, to in-house signs, to a patient view on enduring pain. "We don't do things without consulting these groups," Ms. Wiggins says. "We are trying to have patients or family members on all our hospital committees, including those that deal with medical quality, safety, and performance. We want to be sure we always have the voice of the patient in the room."

In the last six months, Ms. Wiggins says, MMC has adopted a new policy to let family members be present when healthcare providers work to resuscitate a family member. Discharge interviews that include family members have also been designed to give patients a better understanding of the medications they will need to take at home.

In a departure from rigid organizational hierarchies, the nurses, not administration, now make decisions about changed practices. For example, Ms. Wiggins says, the practice council, which is comprised of and chaired by clinical nurses, recently decided that nurses would assess patients and administer influenza vaccines to those who need them. Pulmonologists had emphasized the need to increase vaccination rates. "The nurses decided it was the right thing to do, even though it was more work for them," Ms. Wiggins recalls.

The two CNLs who helped patients and saved money both worked in the Intensive Care Unit. In one instance, they noticed inconsistencies in how different physicians followed the protocol for ventilator care. They collected data and did ventilator rounds every day with physicians, staff, and patients. After finding that some patients were being left on breathing machines longer than necessary, a mutually agreed-upon protocol was implemented. The number of patient days on ventilators was reduced by 18.2 percent over a year's time, and the number of days of intensive care use was reduced by the same amount, saving more than $800,000. In addition, ICU beds were freed up for patients who needed them. "The CNLs' work involved the whole patient care team in the microsystems," Ms. Wiggins says, "and we now have a consistent process in how patients are weaned off the ventilator. And it's best for the patients to be on for just the right amount time, and then get them off."

A CNL also improved patient care after knee surgery. Patients lose a great deal of blood during the surgery, Ms. Wiggins explains, so traditional practice had been to collect the patient's own blood, then re-transfuse it back into the patient. It was a tedious and expensive process that carried some risk. A CNL did a retrospective review of 150 medical records, and discovered no change in the patients' blood counts before and after the procedure. "She went to the orthopedic surgeons and said she realized the practice had been used for some time, but that her evidence showed that in addition to not doing anything good for the patient, the re-transfusions were creating opportunity for infection." The surgeons agreed to eliminate the procedure for knee replacements, the patients were spared the time and risk, and MMC saved more than $150,000 in a year.

"I speak around the country about the CNL role, and I've heard examples like this over and over. In Mobile, Alabama, recently, I heard about a CNL who implemented a process that achieved one-hundred percent elimination of infection in PICC lines (PICC means percutaneous insertion of central catheter). I'm hearing wonderful stories about work being done by CNLs at the microsystem level that are eliminating error and improving quality," Ms. Wiggins says. "I am very satisfied that new roles in nursing, and people who are now educated with a different view of performance will bring a wave of change. And the first wave of change will come from improvements in patient care discovered at this level."

Marjorie S. Wiggins, MBA, RN, NEA-BC, is vice president of nursing and chief nursing officer at Maine Medical Center, Portland. Prior to this she held senior nursing leadership positions in Massachusetts at Beth Israel Deaconess Medical Center and Holy Family Hospital and Medical Center. Ms. Wiggins is highly regarded for her leadership on new patient care delivery models and has written and consulted on these models in the United States and other countries. She played a leading role in developing the Clinical Nurse Leader role through her service on multiple committees of the American Association of Colleges of Nursing. In addition to her nursing leadership work, Ms. Wiggins serves as on the nursing faculty at University of Southern Maine.

Works Cited

1. H. Melvill, 2008. Available from http://www.melvilliana.com/riffs2.htm.

2. "U.S. Health Care Costs," 2008. Available from http://www.kaiseredu.org/topics_im.asp?imID=1&parentID=61&id=358.

3. A. L. Tucker, "Organizational Learning from Operational Failures" (Doctoral Dissertation, Harvard University, 2003).

4. A. L. Tucker and A. C. Edmondson, "Why Hospitals Don't Learn from Failures: Organizational and Psychological Dynamics that Inhibit System Change," Available from http://www.hbs.edu/research/facpubs/workingpapers/papers2/0203/03-059.pdf.

5. J. Begun and K. White, "Altering Nursing's Dominant Logic: Guidelines From Complex Adaptive Systems Theory," *Complexity and Chaos in Nursing* 2, no. 5 (1995): 5-15, 6.

6. Institute of Medicine and Committee on Quality of Healthcare in America, *To Err is Human: Building a Safer Healthcare System for the 21st Century* (Washington D.C.: National Academies Press, 2000).

7. Institute of Medicine and Committee on Quality of Healthcare in America, *Crossing the Quality Chasm: A New Healthcare System for the 21st Century* (Washington D.C.: National Academies Press, 2001).

8. T. Porter-O'grady, "Profound Change: 21st Century Nursing," *Nursing Outlook* 49, no. 4 (2001): 182-186, 183.

9. M. Manthey, *The Practice of Primary Nursing* (Boston: Blackwell Scientific Publications, Inc., 1980).

10. J. Fawcett, *Contemporary Nursing Knowledge: Analysis and Evaluation of Nursing Models and Theories* 2nd ed. (Philadelphia: F.A. Davis, 2005).

11. , *The American Heritage Dictionary of the English Language* 4th ed. (Boston: Houghton Mifflin Co., 2003).

12. J. Holland, *University of Minnesota Conference Proceedings*. 2003.

13. M. S. Wiggins, "The Partnership Care Delivery Model," *Journal of Nursing Administration* 36, no. 78 (2006): 341-345.

14. E. C. Nelson, P. Batalden, and M. M. Godfrey, *Quality by Design: A Microsystems Approach* (San Francisco: John Wiley and Sons, 2007).

15. American Association of Colleges of Nursing, "White Paper on the Education and Role of the Clinical Nurse Leader," 2008. Available from http://www.aacn.nche.edu/Publications/WhitePapers/ClinicalNurseLeader07.pdf.

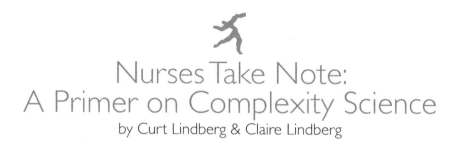

Nurses Take Note:
A Primer on Complexity Science
by Curt Lindberg & Claire Lindberg

We live in a world that is becoming increasing complex. Unfortunately, our style of thinking rarely matches this complexity.[1]

Introduction

This chapter provides an introduction to the concepts and principles of Complexity Science and emphasizes the relevance of Complexity Science to nurses, nursing care, patients, and the healthcare system. Complexity Science is defined, and then explained in terms of its history and interdisciplinary nature. Complex adaptive systems (CASs) are defined and differentiated from traditional, mechanistic viewpoints, and important properties and principles of complex systems are explained and illustrated by examples. The Theory of Complex Responsive Processes is discussed. Insights from Complexity Science particularly applicable to nursing are discussed.

If you are a nurse who has worked in a hospital recently, you will probably identify with Emily's story. Unfortunately, many nurses work in similar conditions. Over the past quarter of a century, the acuity level of hospitalized patients has increased greatly, the technology of care has become increasingly sophisticated, and fiscal exigencies combined with the critical nursing shortage have led to higher nurse-to-patient ratios. While nursing is now once again seen as a desirable career for young men and women, the aging of the nursing workforce combined with high turnover resulting from stress and burnout has left nurses like Emily and Kate working in a highly complex and uncertain situation with few truly experienced mentors.

Research on organizational dynamics and change done in hospital settings demonstrates that during an average eight-hour shift, an RN completes 160 tasks and spends 2.5 minutes on each task.[2] Such fast-paced and demanding work environments have led to medical errors and nurse

A Nurse's Tale

Emily Evans, an RN with two years of nursing experience, arrives to begin her twelve-hour shift on 2E, a busy telemetry unit in St. Jude's Community Hospital. Her assignment includes three patients who are classified as "stable" and one who is classified as "critical." Emily's two years of nursing experience make her one of the most senior nurses on the unit so, she is also assigned to precept Katie Greene, a newly licensed RN. Because Katie is a new graduate and is just completing her initial hospital orientation, her assignment is light. Katie is assigned to care for three patients, each classified as "stable."

When Emily and Katie receive report, they learn that one of Emily's "stable" patients has developed a new cardiac arrhythmia which is potentially life-threatening. His four new medications have not arrived on the floor yet. Another of her "stable" patients is scheduled to go to the OR in two hours, and there are new or-

ders on the chart to carry out for that patient. The third "stable" one is scheduled for discharge but no patient education has been done regarding self-administration of her oral anticoagulant medication. There is nothing new on her critical patient, whom Emily had also cared for on the previous day. Katie's patients include one to be discharged and one recovering well from a quadruple bypass. Her third patient is an eighty-year-old woman with CHF who has a "do not resuscitate (DNR)" order on her chart. This patient's daughter is with her and is providing the patient's personal care. A second daughter, who is a physician, is on her way in from another state to visit. When the report is completed, Emily notices that Katie looks nervous, so she leans over to her and says "It's OK, we can handle this." They set off together to make their rounds. Katie looks visibly relieved to have a preceptor who is so experienced and confident. She is sure that Emily will burnout. It is not surprising that nurses like Emily are frustrated, feel that their workdays are out of control, and worry they are not providing the care patients deserve. Unfortunately, the education provided to nurses today does not prepare them well for working under such stressful conditions or for solving the complex problems they face every day. Nursing education may prepare nurses for facing simple and complicated problems and situations, but simple and complicated problems are different from the complex problems and situations nurses often face today.

According to Glouberman and Zimmerman,[3] simple problems are those that can be solved by following instructions. Glouberman and Zimmerman use the example of following a recipe. In the clinical arena, an example would be following a basic practice protocol. Since simple problems are relatively straightforward, successful resolution is likely when the pre-

help her keep everything under control.

Two hours later, things have begun to unravel on 2E. The medications for Emily's patient who has the arrhythmia have not arrived from the pharmacy and his condition is precarious. Emily has spent much of her time at his bedside trying to keep his condition from deteriorating. His wife is standing by the nurses' station yelling at the unit clerk to "do something to get the medications up here!" The OR has called for Emily's pre-op patient but Emily has not had time to get the orders completed and there is no surgical consent on the chart. The ER has called three times to see if Emily's third patient has gone home. They need the bed for a patient who is ready for transfer to the floor for cardiac monitoring.

Katie's discharge went well, but now she has a new admission. The second daughter of the patient with the DNR order has arrived and the two sisters are loudly arguing about

their mother's care. A few minutes ago, Katie walked into the room to see what was happening, and the physician-daughter began to yell at her. While the two daughters argued, their mother fell out of bed. Katie is now at Emily's side with tears running down her face. "Ok," Emily thinks, "I need some help here now." She looks for the nurse manager and is told that the manager is at an all-day budget meeting and cannot be disturbed and the assistant nurse manager is out sick. Emily realizes that she is on her own. Just at this moment, the cell phone attached to her waist pack rings. It is her husband asking her what he should do—their twelve-month-old has a fever and just vomited up the Tylenol he was given. Emily wonders, for the umpteenth time, whether nursing is the right career choice for her. She vows to talk to her husband about whether they can afford for her to leave her job and go to law school. ■

determined steps are followed. It does not take high levels of expertise to solve simple problems.

Complicated problems are made up of subsets of simple problems. These problems are complicated because they cannot be broken down or reduced to the simple problems they contain. Complicated problems require specialized expertise to solve, but they can be resolved by experts who have high levels of knowledge and experience using or applying pre-existing formulas. Another characteristic of complicated problems is that when the problem is managed by such knowledgeable experts, outcomes can be predicted with a high degree of certainty. In addition, previous successful outcomes with similar problems can be reproduced. The example of a complicated problem presented by Glouberman and Zimmerman is sending a rocket to the moon. Some issues faced by nurses are of this complicated nature, however, many problems and situations faced by nurses are beyond complicated. They are complex.

Table 1: Simple, complicated, and complex problems[23]

Simple	Complicated	Complex
Baking a Cake	Sending a Rocket to the Moon	Raising a Child
The recipe is essential	Rigid protocols or formulas are needed	Rigid protocols have a limited application or are counter-productive
Recipes are tested to assure easy replication	Sending one rocket increases assurance that the next will be a success	Raising a child provides experience but is no guarantee of success with the next
No particular expertise is required, but cooking expertise increases success rate	High levels of expertise and training in a variety of fields are necessary for success	Expertise helps but only when balanced with responsiveness to the particular child
A good recipe produces nearly the same cake every time	Key elements of each rocket MUST be identical to succeed	Every child is unique and must be understood as an individual
The best recipes give good results every time	There is a high degree of certainty of outcome	Uncertainty of outcome remains
A good recipe notes the quantity and nature of the "parts" needed and specifies the order in which to combine them, but there is room for experimentation	Success depends on a blueprint that directs both the development of separate parts and specifies the exact relationship in which to assemble them	Can't separate the parts from the whole; essence exists in the relationship between different people, different experiences, different moments in time

* From Westley, Zimmerman, and Quinn Patton (2006), p. 9

Complex situations display properties of uniqueness, and thus must be approached and understood individually. There is a high degree of uncertainty inherent in complex problems and situations, and outcomes are not predictable. Solutions cannot be assured through application of known formulas. Likewise, expertise and experience are helpful, but do not always insure successful resolution. Complex problems call for unique solutions. The example that Glouberman and Zimmerman use to illustrate a complex problem is raising a child. Nurses today, who are frequently presented with situations that are complex, often do not have the needed knowledge or background. Table 1 describes the attributes of simple, complicated, and complex problems.

In *A Nurse's Tale*, Emily's story illustrates some of the complex issues nurses face at work. Like Emily, most nurses encounter a range of issues during each work shift. Some are complicated, such as balancing the care needs of a small number of patients whose conditions remain stable. Situations such as the ones faced by Emily and Katie, which display the properties of complex problems, are now all too common. For Emily and Katie,

Box A: Examples of complex challenges in nursing

- Caring for patients with multiple chronic diseases
- Helping patients change long-standing habits of unhealthy behavior
- Shaping healthcare policy in a manner that results in better outcomes for patients and communities
- Creating work environments that satisfy and attract nursing personnel
- Preparing healthcare organizations and healthcare systems to cope with emerging infectious diseases
- Designing effective approaches to collaboration with healthcare professionals from different disciplines and within nursing
- Tackling seemingly intractable healthcare quality problems like the spread of deadly antibiotic resistant bacteria, such as MRSA, in hospitals, nursing homes, and communities
- Developing new approaches to learning in nursing schools
- Designing new methods for nursing and healthcare research that match the complexity of the issues being explored
- Establishing new nursing roles

the instability of patients' medical conditions makes it difficult to predict the outcomes of their nursing interventions. Such instability makes it difficult for the nurses to plan care for individual patients. Planning care for multiple patients is exponentially more complex.

Environmental elements also add to the complexity of the problems faced by nurses. Multiple healthcare providers are involved in the care of every patient, necessitating high levels of intra and interdisciplinary collaboration. Patients move between units of care multiple times during a hospital stay and sometimes even during a single day, requiring patient tracking, inter-unit communication, and care coordination to prevent errors during handoffs. Among the many other factors nurses must deal with is the network of family and friends that affect each patient's life. Although not technically part of the healthcare system, these individuals and groups have great potential to increase the complexity of any nurse-patient interaction, as A Nurse's Tale illustrates. Emily's story also demonstrates that working as a staff nurse in a hospital or similar setting is highly complex. Nurses work in many other settings as well, in many differing professional roles, and with varying types of clients. Some additional complex challenges faced by nurses are listed in Box A.

The dominant Newtonian paradigm that underlies most nursing education programs assumes that issues can be understood through careful analysis, rational plans can achieve desired outcomes, and that careful implementation will lead to the expected outcomes.

Current nursing education programs do not go far enough in preparing nurses to work on such complex issues. The dominant Newtonian paradigm that underlies most nursing education programs assumes that most issues can be understood through careful analysis, that rational plans created by experts can achieve desired outcomes, that implementation of plans can be kept on track through regular measurement and feedback, and that careful implementation will lead to the expected outcomes. The Newtonian view dominates the "medical model" which guides much of the healthcare provided in developed nations. The very structure of the predominant healthcare paradigm is one of reductionism. Consider the way patients are viewed as having broken mechanisms or parts (for example, a blocked coronary artery) which can be repaired by doctors specializing in those parts (such as a cardiovascular surgeon). Nursing education prepares nursing students to work within this mechanistically oriented system, and thus most education focuses on linear processes such as developing care plans, implementing specific nursing actions, and expecting predictable and measurable results.

Looking through a historical lens helps to explain this situation. Nursing education developed in an era when nurses were viewed as doctors' "handmaidens" and when the primary causes of death were infection and trauma. Prior to the maturation of modern healthcare with its focus on pharmaceutical treatments and technological advancements, the course of most serious illnesses was rather predictable. Patients got sick and one of two things happened: They recovered after some rest and supportive care or, as was often the case, they died. We now live in a world where, in developed countries, medical science and public health have advanced to the point that many historically predominant causes of death such as smallpox, plague, and community acquired pneumonia are either curable or preventable. The major causes of death are now those related to chronic conditions which have complex bio-behavioral etiologies and variable trajectories. Life ends more slowly in the developed world these days and patients and clinicians cling to it tenaciously, necessitating complex care at the end of life. This is all taking place in a healthcare environment on the brink of disaster because of multiple factors including increased costs related to care and constraints on reimbursement.

In today's complex and uncertain social and healthcare environments, the Newtonian paradigm is rapidly proving insufficient. The Institute of Medicine (IOM) recognized this in its landmark publication, *Crossing the Quality Chasm: A New Health System for the 21st Century*.[4] The IOM cited the shift in healthcare from primarily hospital-based to primarily community-based, increases in the number of patients with chronic multi-system disorders, rapid growth of healthcare technologies, large increases in the healthcare knowledge base, and the explosive growth in the number of pharmaceuticals as forces driving the increased complexity of the healthcare system. The IOM report goes even further in its analysis of the healthcare quality crisis by recognizing that healthcare organizations are CASs and that approaches to addressing quality must recognize this perspective.

By now, you may be asking, "What is a CAS?" The terms *complex* and *system* intuitively make sense to most nurses when they think about the organizations where they work. Many nurses have an understanding of *adaptation* from their studies of biology, evolution, and nursing theory. But what about this term *complex adaptive system* (CAS)? What does it mean and how does it apply to nurses' working environments and the patients under their care? Breaking the term down can lead to a better understanding. *Complex* indicates that the system is composed of numerous, diverse parts, also referred to as *agents*. Agents in the healthcare system include nurses, patients, doctors, family members, pharmaceutical sales representatives, and unit clerks. Examples of agents in biological systems include a molecule, a person, a nursing unit, a cell, a hormone, and an individual plant. *Complex* also recognizes that there are many interactions and relationships among agents within systems. *Adaptive* suggests flexibility, or the ability of agents to learn or change. *System* implies that there are many coordinated elements, or agents, which taken together constitute a whole. In addition, system implies that the elements in the system are interdependent, as well as interactive.[5] CASs are ubiquitous in the biological world and society. Examples include insect colonies, the oceanic ecosystem, communities, families, healthcare systems, nursing care units, and the human body. Within the human body, many systems, such as the neurological and immune systems, also exemplify CASs. CASs are a focus of an emerging interdisciplinary field called Complexity Science.

Complexity Science posits a world-view that is very different from the one inherent in the traditional Newtonian world-view which considers that all things are equal to, but not more than, the sum of their parts and thus can be somewhat cleanly divided into those parts. Think of an engine that can be divided into gears, cams, and other metal parts. This paradigm is called *mechanistic*, in that it assumes that all systems are structured like and behave like machines. Scientists working from a mechanistic perspective seek to gain understanding of an object, process, or relationship, by parsing it into ever smaller and smaller units and studying each of those units separately or in simple combinations. This process of studying the whole by examining the parts is called *reductionism*. Reductionism has been the dominant paradigm underlying research in most scientific fields, including biology, physics, chemistry, sociology, psychology and nursing, for the last century. The dominant research methods used in reductionist science are quantitative. These research methods, which are commonly emphasized in nursing curricula, rely on techniques of measurement and mathematics, using these to calculate outcomes or results of controlled studies. The aims of this type of research are prediction and control.

In contrast, research methods which focus on understanding the lived experiences of individuals and groups through such methods as observation and participant observation, and individual and group interviews are more in keeping with a Complexity Science world-view. These qualitative methodologies, which are earning more respect throughout nursing, medicine, and related fields, are better suited for studying human interactions and perspectives. Multi-method studies which combine qualitative and quantitative methods are also appropriate. Anderson, Crabtree, Steel, and McDaniel[6] propose that a case study design based on a Complexity Science perspective is uniquely suited to help us understand the intricate dynamics in healthcare systems and can lead us to a better understanding of the patterns of relationships and interactions that affect those dynamics. An example of a research study using a theoretical framework derived from Complexity Science is a study of management practices and nursing home resident outcomes by Anderson, Issel, and McDaniel.[7]

Another term used to illustrate the principles of Newtonian science is *clockware*.[5;8] This term conjures up an image of an old-fashioned mechanical clock with its gears, springs, nuts, and bolts. Such simple instruments can be studied by disassembling them and examining the parts. Because the mechanism is simple, the functions of the various parts are easily understood and when the examination is complete, the simple machine can be easily put back together again, returning it to full function. The Newtonian world-view proposes that most things in the world follow the simple principles of clockware.

Another basic assumption of the mechanistic, or Newtonian world-view, is that the function of a unit is influenced by only a limited number of internal or external forces. Thus, it is seen as relatively easy to make predictions about what will happen under a given set of circumstances. This leads to linear ways of thinking, for example, "If I do A, the result will always be B." Because this world-view is based on a machine model, things such as choice, independent decision making, self-determination, and learning are not considered when analyzing actions or behavior. Unpredictability and surprise have no place within this perspective. For example, an experiment that leads to surprising results might be viewed as either fraught with errors or just simply as something that is not yet fully explained.

Mechanistic models cannot be completely disregarded or discarded as many objects and processes in healthcare workplaces generally do exemplify this model. For example, many of the basic instruments used in patient care, such as blood pressure cuffs, thermometers, IV pumps, and oxygen flow meters, were developed within and can be easily understood through this lens. Many straightforward medical procedures can be understood this way as well. Consider treatment of a simple long bone fracture in a healthy, twenty-five-year-old snowboarder in Vermont. The snowboarder falls in December, the fracture is identified and located by X-ray, the orthopedist applies a cast, and the snowboarder heals without any adverse sequeli. He is back on the slopes by March to enjoy the spring snowboarding season. However, despite the fact that the mechanistic model has led to important advances in science and technology—particularly in the physical sciences and engineering—this model is proving to be too simplistic to explain many current phenomena. As the healthcare workplace has become more complex, and scientific understanding of physiologic processes, pathophysiologic processes, and of human systems has expanded, nurses must look to new models, such as Complexity Science, to help explain the phenomena they encounter in their daily work.

Complexity Science is not a single theory, but rather an interdisciplinary field that recognizes multiple theoretical frameworks.

Complexity Science

Complexity Science is not a single theory, but rather an interdisciplinary field that recognizes multiple theoretical frameworks.[5;9] Complexity Science examines systems comprised of multiple and diverse interacting agents and seeks to uncover the principles and dynamics that affect how such systems evolve and maintain order. It is recognized by many as a profoundly important development in science. In an interview with Glennda

Table 2: Selected complexity scientists and their contributions

Scientist	Contributions	Key References
Illya Prigogine Chemist; Winner of Nobel Prize	Discovered that small fluctuations in chemical systems lead to qualitatively different regimes under far from equilibrium conditions	*Order Out of Chaos: Man's New Dialogue with Nature*[24]
Edward O. Wilson Biologist and entomologist; Winner of two Pulitzer Prizes; National Medal of Science and Crafoord Prize	Uncovered self-organizing processes in insect societies First to study role of biodiversity in healthy ecosystems	*The Diversity of Life*[12] *Biodiversity*[25]
Stuart Kauffman Biologist and physician; Winner of MacArthur Award	Developed edge of chaos and order for free concepts Leader in development of Complexity Science	*At Home in the Universe: The Search for Laws of Self-Organization and Complexity*[26] *Reinventing the Sacred: A New View of Science, Reason, and Religion*[27]
Benoit Mandelbrot Mathematician	Developed the concept of fractals and new branch of mathematics called fractal geometry	*The Fractal Geometry of Nature*[28]
Norbert Elias Sociologist	Studied development of complex social networks, societies, and how patterns of behavior arise from ordinary human interactions	*The Society of Individuals*[29] *The Civilizing Process*[30]
Murray Gell-Mann Physicist; Winner of Nobel Prize	Helped found the Santa Fe Institute Conducted early study of CASs	*The Quark and the Jaguar*[31]
Albert-László Barabási Physicist	Led creation of network theory field and developed scale free network concepts	*Linked: The New Science of Networks*[32]
Edward Lorenz Mathematician and meteorologist; Winner of Crafoord Prize	Helped found chaos theory and discovered principle of sensitive dependence on initial conditions	*The Essence of Chaos*[15]
J. Scott Kelso Neuroscientist	Founded field of coordination dynamics—how the body, through self-organizing processes, coordinates movement	*Dynamic Patterns: The Self-Organization of Brain and Behavior*[33]
Ralph Stacey Organizational theorist	Created complexity-informed theory of human organizing called complex responsive processes	*Strategic Management and Organisational Dynamics: The Challenge of Complexity to Ways of Thinking About Organisations*[34]

Chui,[10] physicist and international scholar Stephen Hawking called the twenty-first century "the century of complexity." This young science began its rapid development in the 1980s. At that time, scientists from many disciplines began to notice that discoveries related to system behavior in their fields were similar to discoveries in many other fields. Complexity Science can be viewed as a transdisciplinary field founded by biologists, physicists, economists, neuroscientists, ecologists, chemists, sociologists, computer scientists, and mathematicians. Table 2 presents the work of selected scientists whose scholarship has laid some of the major foundations for this field and provides a sense of both the breadth of the field and the contributions of some important complexity scientists.

A fairly well-known example of a theoretical framework associated with Complexity Science is chaos theory, a body of knowledge used extensively in physics and mathematics. Studies of macrosystems, such as populations or the weather, have been based upon the principles of chaos theory. One tool used by scientists working with chaos theory is complex mathematical modeling.[9] Among other theoretical frameworks or system dynamics generally encompassed by Complexity Science are CASs, nonlinear dynamics, and complex responsive processes (CRPs). The theories of CASs and CRPs are described below. It should be noted that many of the concepts, principles, and terms described in the following two sections are not exclusive to CASs and CRPs, but are commonly encountered throughout Complexity Science.

Complex Adaptive Systems

CASs are a type of complex system with special relevance to nurses and other healthcare professionals. This theory is also being employed widely in the social, biological, and economic sciences. In healthcare, CAS concepts and principles are being tapped in such diverse efforts as prevention of the spread of multi-drug resistant organisms, communications related to HIV/AIDS prevention, nursing workforce issues, optimizing leadership potential, improving patient outcomes in nursing homes, and as a theoretical basis for research on such diverse issues as healthcare quality and the underlying physiologic patterns of chronic diseases. CAS principles are also being used to improve nursing education.

CASs are *dynamic*. In the more traditional view of systems, posited by *General Systems Theory*,[11] systems are viewed as adaptable but with the goal of stability. In general systems theory, systems are seen as striving to fend off change in order to maintain an *equilibrium* or steady state. According to general systems theory, a system which loses its ability to maintain equilibrium will cease to exist. In contrast, according to the theory of CASs, a healthy system is always poised to change. A system without this dynamic capacity cannot survive.

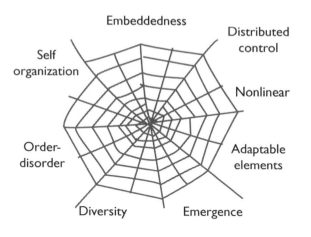

Figure 1: Properties of complex adaptive systems

To further understand CASs it is helpful to consider the major properties of such systems which include diversity, self-organization, embeddedness, distributed control, nonlinear dynamics, adaptable elements, emergence, and the coexistence of order and disorder. Figure 1 illustrates how these key properties are interrelated by placing them on a web.

As described above, CASs are made up of many *interconnected, interdependent, adaptive*, and *diverse* elements. Diversity enables the system to adapt or change when confronted with a challenge. We have all experienced change triggered by a new idea introduced into a conversation or the view of professionals from another field and the difference it can make in facing a complex patient challenge. New insights and ways forward may emerge when diverse voices are welcomed. Biologist Edward O. Wilson demonstrated that diversity is an essential ingredient in healthy ecosystems.[12] Wilson writes in *The Creation* that each species, "however humble and inconspicuous it may seem to us at this moment, is a masterpiece of biology and well worth saving."[13] He maintains that the healthiest environmental systems are teeming with diverse species, and that civilizations collapse when their environments are ruined.

A related CAS property is *embeddedness*. Each agent in a CAS is, in it-self, a CAS, and is in turn made up of other CASs. Thus, every CAS is *embedded* in a larger CAS. To understand this principle, think of a nurse who is an individual CAS and also an agent within other CASs. The nurse is embedded in a nursing unit, which is embedded in a hospital, which is embedded in a local healthcare system, which is embedded in a commu-nity, and so on. Embeddedness matters because each CAS shapes and is simultaneously shaped by interactions with other CASs. Complexity sci-entists call this mutual shaping co-evolution. This emphasis on the mutual effects of interactions between agents and systems contrasts with a com-mon subtext of conversations heard in the hallways and cafeterias of many organizations: "I am an insignificant cog (notice the machine metaphor) in the system. It doesn't matter what I do or say, nothing will change." In fact, every action by every person matters and in turn affects everything and everybody else.

The principle of co-evolution recognizes that even a small change in a single element within a single system can have an impact on the larger whole. For example, in the situation on Unit 2E described above, the dis-ruption in Emily's routine caused by the pharmacy's failure to deliver her patient's medications leads to her inability to devote time to her other pa-tients' needs, which in turn leads to repercussions for her other patients, for the OR staff, the ER staff, Katie, and Katie's patients.

Within CASs, control is shared by many agents, rather than being cen-tralized. This property, known as *distributed control*, allows the system to reap the benefits of diversity. An example might be seen in considering the difference between two hospital units. Unit A is run by Sarah Kaplan, a bright, well-meaning, and experienced nurse manager who has learned traditional management methods. While Sarah always listens to the ideas and concerns of her staff, she maintains the prerogative to make all final decisions. She tends to feel threatened by new ideas and discards those that differ from her own. Sarah believes that change must be directed, that order must be maintained, and that because she is the designated leader, she probably knows best how to solve the problems her staff encounters.

Although the demands of patient care on Unit A have changed drasti-cally over time, little has changed in the way care is delivered, largely be-cause of the attitude of the nurse manager. The unit staff, although they like their manager personally, are frustrated and feels overworked and unengaged. It is common for staff to suffer from burnout and consequently staff turnover is high. Patient satisfaction is relatively low. Contrast the situation on Unit A with the situation on Unit B. Unit B is run by Lisa Crane, a nurse manager who has been in the job only two years and who learned principles of complexity in her graduate nursing program. Lisa not only listens to her staff, she encourages them to collaborate to solve problems and to develop new methods of patient care delivery. The diversity of expressed ideas and active communication on the unit resulted in quite a few advances in the way care is delivered. The atmosphere on this unit is one of collaboration and cooperation. Quite to the surprise of the professional nursing staff, many excellent ideas have originated with the nursing assistants, unit secretaries, and housekeeping staff. There has been no turnover in nursing staff in the two years she has managed the unit, and patient safety and satisfaction have improved. One can see that Lisa understands the value of diversity and the principle of *distributed control* and has tapped into the power of the unit. She recognizes the limitations of a view that honors stability as the prime goal and understands that in healthy CASs, *order* and *disorder* coexist. Lisa was first introduced to these concepts in her advanced pathophysiology course where she learned that the healthy cardiovascular system in a young adult exhibits both regularity and variability at the same time. This dynamic, termed *edge of chaos* or *far from equilibrium*, is found in many systems when they are at their most adaptable. She read that the loss of complexity—too much regularity or too much variability—is associated with many unhealthy conditions like congestive heart failure and atrial fibrillation.

Distributed control may be intentional, but even when it is not intentional, it is a powerful force within an organization. In an organization with a rigid, formal hierarchy of authority, the ideas and creativity of the average worker may not be sought or acknowledged. While the ideas of these workers may be formally disregarded, their influence cannot be eliminated. Hence, control is still distributed even though it is not understood as such. Workers without authority can influence the outcomes of management initiatives through active support or active or passive resistance and thus can be a powerful element in any organizational system. This informal network is sometimes referred to as the "shadow system."[14] Within the shadow system there are informal power figures and thought leaders who can influence activities within that system. Effective managers learn to understand the shadow system and appreciate its impact on the organization. Most nurses can think of examples wherein the formal hospital authority system decreed that a new policy or other change should be implemented, only to find that it is not carried out on one or more units. This scenario is often caused by resistance that originates in the shadow system. A major point illustrated by the principle of distributed control is that no one, no matter how wise or powerful, is able to control outcomes in self-organizing complex systems.

CASs are open to influence from multiple forces from within and from outside. The forces and interactions within and between systems may lead to the creation of novel patterns, structures, and processes through a process called *self-organization*. Before this concept was understood, many theorists informed by traditional systems theory believed that systems, once disturbed, tried to return to a prior state called equilibrium or one of

Box B: An example of self-organization

And Extraordinary Day in Labor and Delivery

When Janet Kramer BS, RN clocked in for her twelve-hour shift as charge nurse on the labor and delivery (L&D) unit, things on the unit looked fairly quiet. There were only three women in labor. Staffing looked adequate. Janet and two other RNs were assigned to the unit along with two aides. The staff looked forward to having some time to organize the unit stock room and complete some standardized care plans and policies that were requested by the unit nurse manager in anticipation of a Joint Commission visit.

The Clinical Nurse Leader® from the post-partum unit stopped by early in the shift to check on the status of the laboring moms so she could anticipate her unit's needs. Janet's assigned patient delivered a seven-pound-eight-ounce baby girl early in the shift and was transferred quickly to post-partum. Now the unit only had two patients, both in early labor. Janet agreed that the two aides could go to the nursery to help with infant care. One RN went to dinner and Janet sat down to look over the policy on nursing management of patients having preterm labor. At this point, the phone rang. It was the ER advising her that they were transferring up a thirteen-year-old in labor who had not known she was pregnant. They tell Janet that the girl's mother is close to hysterical.

As Janet readied a bed for the girl, the phone rang again. It was the antepartum unit advising her that they were sending a patient pregnant with triplets back to L&D. As soon as she put down the phone, it rang again. It was Dr. Flores, advising her that she was sending in a woman in labor who had a history of pre-eclampsia and that she anticipated doing a C-section within the next few hours. Within the next hour, the several predetermined states called archetypes. In nursing, as well as in medicine, biology, and physiology, this equilibrium or "steady state" is referred to as "homeostasis." An implication of the traditional view is that change is a negative force which must be resisted or overcome with the goal of maintaining the status quo. In contrast, the theory of CASs recognizes both the inevitable nature and positive and negative aspects of the self-organizing process. This process is governed by interactions among the diverse elements of the CAS. A story that illustrates the principles of self-organization and distributed control in relationship to a complex and potentially disastrous situation on a mother-baby unit can be found in Box B.

The result of self-organizing processes may be evolution to a completely novel state. Scientists term the outcome of self-organizing processes emergence. An example of emergence in the story in Box B include the new staffing patterns that developed in the face of rapidly changing con-

census in L&D goes up to nine patients. Three patients have complex medical issues and one, the teenager, has complex social and psychological needs. Janet anticipated a crisis situation regarding staffing the unit and she knew she needed to call the nurse manager to request additional help. However, she was unable to leave the room where she is trying to stabilize the mother of the triplets. Her concern for the other patients and for the single RN left managing the remaining eight patients was extreme by the time she was able to walk to the nurses station.

What she finds when she leaves the room surprises and relieves her. The RN who was at dinner had a "feeling she should come back up" and cut her dinner short. She is now managing two of the patients. The Clinical Nurse Leader from the postpartum unit has sent over an RN to provide care to two other patients. Dr. Flores, who used to be an L&D

nurse, saw how busy the nurses were when she arrived on the floor and called the head nurse to get a backup team from the main OR to help with the C-section, which is in progress. The two aides, hearing that L&D was busy, came back immediately from the nursery and are tending to the two remaining patients who are both in early labor. One of the aides ran into the unit social work professional as she walked back from the nursery and advised her that there was a thirteen-year-old in early labor. The social worker immediately had come to L&D and was calming down the teenager and her frantic mom. The unit, while busy, is running smoothly and all patient care needs are being met. The well-trained mother-baby team, has self-organized to meet the needs of the laboring mothers by shifting staffing patterns to focus on the unit and patients most in need. ∎

Box C: Examples of emergence

- The onset and remission of a chronic disease
- Life on earth
- An "ah ha" experience when a new insight arose in your mind or in group conversation
- Staph aureus becoming resistant to antibiotics
- The start and course of a war
- Learning that takes place in college nursing courses as students and faculty interact
- A presidential candidate who comes out of the blue
- The emergence of a new species
- Global climate change

ditions on the L&D unit. These staffing patterns were not planned, nor were they predictable at the beginning of the shift. Some other examples of emergence are listed in Box C.

The results of self-organizing processes can never be predicted with certainty. This characteristic unpredictability stems from the multiple, interacting, diverse, and changing elements in the system. Another factor leading to the inability to predict outcomes is the ability of a small change in one of the agents or in the interactions among the agents to ripple through the system and cause a large change. Such disproportionate effects illustrate the principle of *nonlinearity*. Traditional science has long held that the world is composed of linear relationships, those in which a change in A leads to a change in B that is predictable in size and direction. In contrast, nonlinearity implies unpredictability wherein small changes can lead to large effects and vice versa. Surprise is thus an inherent feature of complex systems.

Weather systems are often used to explain the concept of nonlinearity. Many people wonder why it is difficult to predict the weather despite massive computer modeling and sophisticated monitoring systems. Edward Lorenz, a meteorologist at MIT, studied models of atmospheric convection and learned that relationships between initial conditions and resulting weather patterns were nonlinear. In his models, seemingly inconsequential differences in the initial variables led to radically different outcomes.

He expressed this concept in a famous talk titled "Does the flap of a butterfly's wings in Brazil set off a tornado in Texas?" In his remarks, Lorenz hypothesized that a small event, like the beating of a butterfly's wings, could lead to large meteorological effects many miles away,[15] hence the birth of the popularized term the "butterfly effect," used generally to express the central concept of nonlinearity that small changes can lead to large effects.

Complex Responsive Processes

As can be seen from the above discussion, interactions are an essential dynamic in CASs. Organizational theorist Ralph Stacey developed a complexity-informed theory that focuses exclusively on people, and places human interactions in the forefront. In his theory of complex responsive processes, Stacey proposes that processes of human relating create, through self-organization, patterns of interaction that may lead to wide-spread or global patterns of behavior and interaction.[9;16;17] In Stacey's view, a family or nursing unit are not considered CASs, but are instead patterns of interaction that affect and are affected by each participating individual. He states:

> In human process terms, there are no forces [systems] over and above individuals. All we have are vast numbers of iterated interactions and these are local in the sense that each of us can only interact with a limited number of others...[18]

Because these patterns are actively maintained in how we interact in routine, everyday conversations, they simultaneously hold the potential for continuity and change. We have all experienced conversations or other interactions with friends, family members, or colleagues where we can reasonably predict what comes next because it has happened before. We have also experienced conversations that are more free-flowing, where a starting comment caroms around and leads to a whole new stream of ideas. Stacey would observe that the latter conversation or pattern of relating is complex. According to Stacey and Griffin, "Patterns of relating that lose this complexity become rapidly inappropriate for dealing with the fluidity of ordinary, everyday life."[18] These patterns of interacting, be they repetitive or creative and generative, are difficult for us to see because they are taken for granted and seem to have a life of their own. Many times we do not appreciate the role we play in creating them. According to sociologist Norbert Elias:

> ...the basic tissue resulting from many single plans and actions of man can give rise to change and patterns that no individual person has planned or created. From the interdependence of people arises an order *sui generis*, an order more compelling and stronger than the will and reason of the individual people composing it.[19]

According to the theory of CRP, if it is change we are after, and when we see the patterns and our role in their creation, we can make different choices in how we participate in a conversation. Changing how we interact or doing something different in the moment, raise the potential for conflict and anxiety because one cannot know in advance how others will react to our different move. In complexity terms, this introduction of diversity into a pattern of interacting may represent the small change that triggers an entirely new pattern of relating or meaning. This emergence happens through a self-organizing process we can influence but not control. This self-organization is happening all around us and we are active players. One of us wrote:

> ...the essence of organization is common, everyday micro interactions, which entail conflict, difference and uncertain outcomes. The possibility of creating different dynamics at the organization level [such as families, nursing units, classrooms], or what Stacey calls global patterns, can only occur if different patterns emerge from local everyday conversations and actions.[20]

The theory of CRP resonates with nurses because of their theoretical and experiential background in human caring and intimate relationships with patients and families. Family nursing theorists Gweneth Hartrick Doane and Colleen Varcoe advance a Complexity Science-based nursing framework that recognizes the key formative role of relationships.[21] Similar to Stacey's belief in the importance of human interactions, Hartwick Doane & Varcoe consider that all people are products of relational interactions which shape their beliefs, attitudes, structures, identities, values, cultures, knowing, and indeed all their ways of being in the world. The work of Hartwick, Doane, & Varcoe provides practical guidance on how to integrate Complexity Science principles in general, and in particular, relational processes and skills into a type of nursing practice that is collaborative, healing, empowering to nurses, patients, and families, and simultaneously humbling.

With self-organization and emergence in mind, healthcare professionals appreciate that while results of their actions can never be predicted, they always hold the potential for triggering significant change.

CRP theory is also being promoted in the broader healthcare arena. For example, Anthony Suchman has used the theory of complex responsive processes to advance the development of the relationship-centered care model.[22] This model, like that proposed by Hartwick Doane, & Varcoe, emphasizes the importance of relationships as a core principle for humane and effective healthcare.

Closing Thoughts

This chapter has presented some core concepts of Complexity Science and related models and theories, and has discussed their relevance to nursing and healthcare. The implications of these theories for nursing, health, and healthcare are profound. Viewing the world through the lens of Complexity Science provides us with new insights into the complex healthcare system we work within, on the patients, families, and colleagues we interact with, and also on ourselves personally and professionally. Nurses and other healthcare professionals who grow to understand the general features of

Complexity Science and in particular those of CASs and CRP, many times realize that their actions and interactions matter more than they knew. Awareness of complexity concepts thus invites active participation and generates a sense of empowerment and hopefulness. With self-organization and emergence in mind, healthcare professionals appreciate that while results of their actions can never be predicted, they always hold the potential for triggering significant change.

While Complexity Science is considered a relatively young science and its applications to nursing, health, and healthcare are just being discovered, nursing has long embraced some of the key Complexity Science tenets and principles. In fact, Florence Nightingale may have been the first nurse to use some Complexity Science principles in her art and science. Nightingale is widely credited as being the first nurse to study and reach an understanding of the interactive effects of environment, hygiene, nutrition, and nursing actions on health and survival. Nursing is itself a complex profession and our history recognizes the complexity involved in nursing care.

In our work within the nursing community, we have noticed that many nurses have an intuitive sense for Complexity Science. Its principles resonate with nurses because of their exposure to the biological sciences, their experience with patients and families, and most important, their understanding of the central place of interactions and relationships in the healing arts. Nurses have learned to live with uncertainty involved in patient care, to understand that control is an illusion, and to recognize that the many interacting factors that affect the health and well-being of patients and families regularly produce surprises. Many nurses, upon learning about Complexity Science, feel as though their experience, knowledge, and intuitive understanding are being given both structure and voice. These understandings position the nursing profession to lead the introduction and further development of Complexity Science principles into healthcare.

Claire Lindberg, PhD, RN, is a professor of nursing at The College of New Jersey, School of Nursing, Exercise and Health Science where she was responsible for integrating Complexity Science into the graduate nursing curriculum. Dr. Lindberg co-chairs the Nursing and Complexity Network of Plexus Institute. She teaches courses in family nursing, evidence-based practice, and primary care and integrates Complexity Science principles and learning strategies inspired by Complexity Science into her teaching. Dr. Lindberg is a family nurse practitioner with specialties in adolescent medicine and women's health. Her scholarly interests include Complexity Science, health promotion, and HIV/AIDS prevention and care.

Curt Lindberg, DMan, is president of Plexus Institute, an organization devoted to helping people use insights from Complexity Science. Dr. Lindberg has devoted a significant portion of his professional life to bringing Complexity Science insights and complexity-informed practices to the fields of management and healthcare. He has accomplished this through his writing, speaking, and by connecting complexity scientists with organizational and healthcare practitioners. He co-authored the first book devoted to complexity and healthcare: *Edgeware: Insights from Complexity Science for Health Care Leaders*. He holds a doctoral degree in complexity and organizational change from the University of Hertfordshire where he studied under Ralph Stacey.

Works Cited

1. G. Morgan, *Images of Organization* (Thousand Oaks: Sage, 1997), 16.

2. A. L. Tucker, "Organizational Learning from Operational Failures" (Doctoral Dissertation, Harvard University, 2003).

3. S. Glouberman and B. Zimmerman, "Complicated and Complex Systems: What Would Successful Reform of Medicare Look Like?," 2007. Available from http://www.change-ability.ca/publications.html.

4. Institute of Medicine and Committee on Quality of Healthcare in America, *Crossing the Quality Chasm: A New Healthcare System for the 21st Century* (Washington D.C.: National Academies Press, 2001).

5. B. Zimmerman, C. Lindberg, and P. Plsek, *Edgeware: Insights from Complexity Science for Health Care Leaders* (Irving: VHA Inc., 2001).

6. R. A. Anderson et al., "Case Study Research: The View From Complexity Science," *Qualitative Health Research* 15, no. 5 (2005): 669-685.

7. R. A. Anderson, L. M. Issel, and R. R. McDaniel, "Nursing Homes As Complex Adaptive Systems: Relationship Between Management Practice and Resident Outcomes," *Nursing Research* 52, no. 1 (2003): 12-21, 13.

8. K. Kelly, *Out of Control: The New Biology of Machines, Social Systems, and the Economic World* (Reading: Addison Wesley Longman, 1995).

9. R. Stacey, *Complexity and Group Processes: A Radically Social Understanding of Individuals* (Hove: Brunner-Routledge, 2003).

10. G. Chui, "Unified Theory" is Getting Closer, Hawking predicts," *San Jose Mercury News*, 2000, sec. A.

11. L. Von Bertalanffy, "The Theory of Open Systems in Physics and Biology," *Science* 111 (1950): 23-28.

12. E. Wilson, *The Diversity of Life* (Cambridge: The Belknap Press, 1992).

13. E. Wilson, *The Creation: An Appeal to Save Life on Earth* (New York: W.W. Norton, 2006), 4-5.

14. R. Stacey, *Complexity and Creativity in Organizations* (San Francisco: Berrett-Kohler Publishers, 1996).

15. E. Lorenze, *The Essence of Chaos* (London: UCL Press, 1995).

16. R. Stacey, *Complex Responsive Processes in Organizations: Learning and Knowledge Creation* (London: Routledge, 2001).

17. R. Stacey, *Strategic Management and Organisational Dynamics: The Challenge of Complexity to Ways of Thinking* 5 ed. (London: Pearson Education, 2007).

18. R. Stacey and D. Griffin, *A Complexity Perspective on Researching Organizations: Taking Experience Seriously* (London: Routledge, 2005), 18, 7.

19. N. Elias, *On Civilization, Power, and Knowledge* (Chicago: The University of Chicago Press, 1998), 50.

20. C. Lindberg, "Leading Volunteers: Power Relations and Values in Organizations" (Doctoral Dissertation, University of Hertfordshire, Complexity and Management Centre, 2007), 155.

21. G. Hartick Doane and C. Varcoe, *Family Nursing as Relational Inquiry: Developing Health-Promoting Practice* (Philadelphia: Lippincott, Williams & Wilkins, 2005), 52.

22. A. Suchman, "A New Theoretical Foundation for Relationship-Centered Care: Complex Responsive Processes of Relating," *Journal of General Internal Medicine* 21 (2006): 40-44.

23. F. Westley, B. Zimmerman, and M. Quinn Patton, *Getting to Maybe: How the World is Changed* (Mississauga: Random House Canada, 2006), 9.

24. I. Prigogine and I. Stengers, *Order Out of Chaos: Man's New Dialogue with Nature* (New York: Bantam Books, 1984).

25. E. Wilson and P. Francis, *Biodiversity* (Washington, D.C.: National Academy of Sciences, 1996).

26. S. Kauffman, *At Home in the Universe: The Search for Laws of Self-Organization* (New York: Oxford University Press, 1995), 15.

27. S. Kauffman, *Reinventing the Sacred: A New View of Science, Reason, and Religion* (New York: Basic Books, 2008).

28. B. B. Mandelbrot, *The Fractal Geometry of Nature* (San Francisco: W.H. Freeman and Co., 1982).

29. N. Elias, *The Society of Individuals* (New York: Continuum, 2001).

30. N. Elias, *The Civilizing Process: Sociogenetic and Psychogenetic Investigations* (Oxford: Blackwell Publishers, 2000).

31. M. Gell-Man, *The Quark and the Jaguar* (New York: W.H. Freeman and Company, 1994).

32. A. L. Barabasi, *Linked: The New Science of Networks* (Cambridge: Perseus, 2002), 43.

33. J. Kelso, *Dynamic Patterns: The Self-Organization of Brain and Behavior* (Cambridge: MIT Press, 1995).

34. R. Stacey, *Strategic Management and Organisational Dynamics: The Challenge of Complexity to Ways of Thinking* 5 ed. (London: Pearson Education, 2007).

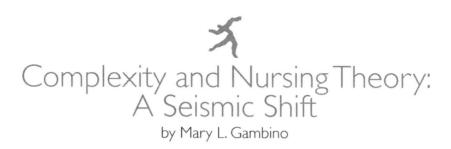

Complexity and Nursing Theory:
A Seismic Shift
by Mary L. Gambino

...the gods have fled.[1]

How do nurses make sense of what they experience in caring for patients and their loved ones? Is there a good way to organize nursing experiences and knowledge to better assist nurses to provide the best possible care? What do nurses do when their experience, knowledge, critical thinking, problem solving, and rational decision making processes are not sufficient for solving the complex problems they face? These are the daily dilemmas that face nurses providing direct patient care, as well as nurses that lead and manage the provision of nursing care. Janice Morse asserted that nursing theories must authentically reflect and provide guidance to the practice of nursing.[2] Nurses are educated to believe that they should be able to derive the answers to these questions from nursing theories or that they should develop new theories from their practice experience, but something is seriously amiss.

Que sais-je? (What do I know?) Montaigne[3]

The twentieth century brought many significant changes in nursing science and nursing practice, and these changes significantly affect the utility of nursing theory. Shirley M. Ziegler, nurse educator and author, recently noted that theory and practice have different purposes, and that one does not necessarily lead to the other—a nuance not necessarily evident in the nursing literature. While theory traditionally describes, explains, or predicts a phenomenon of interest, practice is about the practical use of our understandings to bring about desired changes in the patient or in the care setting. Ziegler suggests there is a need for strategy to connect theory and practice because:

- Rarely do nurses face a nursing situation that consists of a single problem. Rather, nurses face many problems on many levels.

- Problems have more than a single solution.

- Clinical decisions are difficult and outcomes are uncertain.

- Nurses are constantly making choices. These choices are often based on too little knowledge and involve guessing (hypothesizing) about the outcomes of nursing actions. These guesses are most valid if based on theory that has been supported by research.

- Nursing actions, even if based on theory and research, are still creative acts.[4]

Thomas Kuhn[5] identified a phenomenon that is relevant to nursing science today. When a theory in use no longer fits the experiences and observations of the scientists in a field, a scientific revolution will occur. As the detachment of nursing theories from nursing practice grows, fueled by the complexity of care and care giving that Ziegler[4] describes, nursing science will experience a scientific revolution. Pascale, Millemann, and Gioja declare that a "new scientific renaissance [is] in the making,"[6] and nursing—like many other sciences—is already situated in the crosshairs of this renaissance.

Concurrent with this renaissance is the emergence of a new paradigm called Complexity Science. The purpose of this chapter is to promote a better understanding of this scientific renaissance and its relationship to the future of nursing theory, nursing theory development, and most important, the science on which we will base our nursing practice. This renaissance will compel a reexamination of both the philosophy of nursing science and the underlying assumptions about ways of knowing and decision making in patient care, which in turn forms the basis of nursing theory development. The following sections will describe the relationship of Complexity Science to inquiry. They will also address alternative frameworks to Complexity Science, early evidence of the failure of the alternative views of inquiry, and the relationship of Complexity Science to nursing theory while considering Montaigne's philosophical question—*Que sais-je?*

Complexity Science: A Framework for Inquiry

Just over a decade ago, noted nurse theorist and educator Pamela G. Reed[1] published an article on nursing knowledge development for the twenty-first century. In this classic article, Reed noted that important changes were taking place in nursing science relative to the evolving philosophy of science, and that these changes would influence how we thought about theory in the future. Reed predicted that modernism and postmodern thought would lead to the demise of twentieth century theorizing in nursing and to exciting new possibilities in knowledge development.

Nursing is not alone in the scientific renaissance that is occurring across professions. Most professions—like those in healthcare—have become increasingly specialized. Along with specialization comes increased complexity and the need for interdisciplinary collaboration to manage this complexity. Julie Klein,[7] an author and educator in the subjects of humanities and interdisciplinary studies, describes the challenge of interdisciplinarity and the required response of working with problems that are neither predictable nor simple. Managing complex relationships is at the heart of interdisciplinary interaction. Multi-dimensional and ambiguous, systems made up of human beings reflect the values and agendas of all. The recognition is that these interactions are "messy" and resist management by typical problem solving approaches.[7;8] Klein[7] contends that the art of being a professional is becoming the art of managing complexity.

Patient care and management problems faced by nurses today are exactly those that Klein[7] and Ziegler[4] describe. The challenge of responding appropriately to this uncertainty is augmented by a commonly held underlying assumption that knowledge and actions are linear in nature. Such assumptions are shared by a majority of nursing administrators, educators, and scientists. The expectation of linearity, which underlies the current statistical methods used to test theory, exacerbates the incongruence between early nursing theory grounded in biological sciences and nursing practice.

Nurses in practice have long known that linear thinking does not reflect the intricate web of interactions embedded in patient care.

Nurses in practice have long known that linear thinking does not reflect the intricate web of interactions embedded in patient care. Additionally, nurses also understood what Parker Palmer, a well-known educational activist, recognized—we are actually helped, not hindered, by being enmeshed in this web.[9] Philosopher Thomas Kuhn noted that the ability to perceive or "see" something requires use of the right metaphor.[5] The assumptions underlying Complexity Science encompass a nonlinear approach to problem solving that could provide the strategy to bond nursing theory to nursing practice in these uncertain situations.

Pascale et al.[6] considered Complexity Science to be a framework for inquiry. The Complexity Science paradigm fosters a nonlinear world-view, which is what gives Complexity Science its inherent ability to inform a nursing theory renaissance. Complexity Science provides the needed strategy for linking nursing theory and practice by removing the limitations imposed by using primarily linear approaches to problem solving. Complexity Science, as a new world-view, holds promise for being what Kuhn refers to as the right metaphor.

It is only in the past decade that individuals interested in organizations and healthcare began to use Complexity Science to frame research studies in new ways that have significant potential for advancing our understanding of how best to promote the delivery of high-quality, cost-effective care. Recently, Ruth Anderson and colleagues provided the first in-depth explanation of how this framework for nursing inquiry differs from the Newtonian or analytical framework, using examples from their case study research in nursing homes.[10] To achieve a better understanding of why Complexity Science provides a framework for inquiry that is so revolutionary requires some history on the philosophy of science and its impact on nursing theory development.

In the Beginning: The Mechanistic Framework for Inquiry

In *Complexity: The Emerging Science at the Edge of Order*, M. Mitchell Waldrop[11] describes the history of the Santa Fe Institute as instrumental in pioneering Complexity Science. An excerpt from this enlightening account of our changing world-views which is shown in Box A describes how science works, not by deduction, but mainly through metaphors that change over time. This account is based on a conversation with Brian Arthur, an economist with the Institute.

This mechanistic and extremely powerful metaphor of inquiry which began with Newton dominated science for two-and-a-half centuries and was eventually dubbed *clockwork*. Paradigm paralysis[5] took over people's

Box A: An excerpt from
Complexity: The Emerging Science at the Edge of Order (Waldrop, 1992)

Before the seventeenth century, it was a world of trees, disease, human psyche, and human behavior. It was messy and organic. The heavens were also complex. The trajectories of the planets seemed arbitrary. Trying to figure out what was going on in the world was a matter of art. But then along comes Newton in the 1660s. He devises a few laws, he devises the differential calculus—and suddenly the planets are seen to be moving in simple, predictable orbits!

This had an incredible profound effect on people's psyche, right up to the present. The heavens—the habitat of God—had been explained, and you didn't need angels to push things around anymore. You didn't need God to hold things in place.[11] ∎

thinking and locked the world into this mechanistic world-view. What Newtonian physics provided was a reductionistic framework that led scientists and others to believe that the world and its complexity could be, like the predictable clockwork motion of the planets, reduced to a few simple laws. Philosophers and scientists alike used this framework to develop processes and methods based on the assumption that when something was

Box B: History and philosophy of science: key terms and definitions[37]

Empiricism
A theoretical perspective that holds that knowledge is advanced by systematic study and verification of objective observations and experimental methods.

Hypothetico-Deductive Model
The model of science that includes theoretical explanation, hypothesis formation, and hypothesis testing by experimentation.

Logical Positivism
A theoretical perspective that aimed to bring the logic and precision of mathematics to scientific inquiry. Logical Positivism asserted that the only valid approaches to knowledge and truth were logic and the experimental method.

Mechanistic
A theoretical perspective that holds that all natural phenomenon can be explained in terms of physical causes.

Metaparadigm
Refers to the subject matter of most importance to members of a discipline. In nursing, used to describe the four concepts of *man, society, health,* and *nursing,* which are universally accepted as being the major phenomena of interest in the field.

Modernism
Refers to the overall cultural, social, artistic, and scientific context of the Western world. In terms of philosophy of science, modernism refers to the age of scientific discovery and experimentation.

Paradigm
Refers to world-views, defined as patterns or systems of beliefs about science and knowledge production that cross disciplinary boundaries. The paradigm of a discipline determines acceptable views, theories, and scientific methods.

Post-Modernism
A mindset that recognizes the existence of multiple truths or realities and encourages openness to ideas and valuing ideas that include such things as context, stories, narratives, multiple meanings, and realities and wholeness.

Rationalism
A theoretical perspective that posits that reason is, in itself, a superior source of knowledge and is independent of sense perceptions.[50]

Received View
Refers to a philosophical world-view that is generally accepted to be true without criticism. This term is often used to refer to logical positivism.

Reductionism
Refers to theories and beliefs that complex phenomena can be taken apart (reduced) to their component parts. ∎

too complex to understand, the analytical method could be used to divide the entity into units for analysis and then, like a machine, be reassembled.[12] The power of the mechanistic metaphor blinded researchers, educators, and administrators alike to a world-view comprised of a dynamic and intricate web of complex relationships. Box B includes definitions of key terms related to the philosophy and history of science which are used in this chapter.

The mechanistic world-view that arose from these clockwork ideas had a significant influence on nursing science development.[13] As the mechanistic world-view ascended in popularity, there was a nearly forty-year period in philosophy of science known as logical positivism. In the 1960s, this philosophy of science coincided with a movement to develop nursing theory and advance nursing science. Doctoral

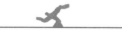

The mechanistic world-view that arose from these clockwork ideas had a significant influence on nursing science development.

preparation of nurse scientists, primarily in the biological sciences, ensued. Therefore, early doctoral training for nurses was grounded in the reductionistic model of inquiry, and the majority of future nurse leaders became grounded in a positivistic, quantitative scientific paradigm. The result was a league of nurse leaders, researchers, and educators with a markedly linear and mechanistic world-view. According to Reed,[1] these nurse researchers linked theory and research through systems of inquiry designed to keep research separate from values, religion, and philosophy. As a result, the reductionistic framework for understanding how things worked became pervasive in nursing theory development.

Rodgers[13] points out that the accepted basis for nursing science and knowledge was grounded on the Newtonian framework for inquiry and framed using empirical data and quantitative research for the purpose of controlling, explaining, and predicting events. This hypotheticodeductive model of research became the accepted method of theory development and testing. The hypotheticodeductive model is a cumulative, linear model, founded on the belief that reality is something that simply exists to be discovered. Reality specific to a particular phenomenon can be understood or explained by studying the parts without the observer's actions affecting the findings. Facts are considered autonomous, unrelated to other facts and their context, and are accumulated and used to build a whole. It is this belief in the ability to reduce the whole into parts that became the main characteristic of the received view during the modernist period and continues to inform experimental and quasi-experimental research methods today. The most important contribution of this reductionistic movement was a concerted effort to examine nursing's knowledge base, thus initiating the development of nursing as a discipline with a separate and distinct body of knowledge.[14]

In the early 1980s, some in nursing began to recognize that the received view held by early nurse theorists had serious limitations in real life application. Rodgers contends that the allegiance of nursing to other disciplines through their early doctoral training, coupled with the lack of awareness of alternative and broader views, helped perpetuate the logical positivism underpinning of nursing theory development. Researchers found themselves unable to overcome the significant limitations imposed by its impossible goals. Perhaps most onerous was the empirical data requirement for studying many phenomena of interest. This requirement created quite a conundrum for researchers interested in multifaceted concepts like hope, dignity, and collaboration. In developing valid and reliable instruments to measure such constructs, a plethora of valid concerns arose about whether any instrument could adequately measure the complexity integral to human experiences and interactions. The linear, cumulative nature of inquiry constrained nursing science development and resulted in a context that left little room for the creativity needed to advance nursing science.[13]

In the following example, note how the underlying tenets of logical positivism created an irreconcilable analysis problem. As early as the 1970s, nurse researchers Hegyvary and Chamings[15] reported on a quasi-experimental study that examined facts exclusive of their context, as was the expectation of good science during this time. The investigators in this study assigned eighty-nine abdominal hysterectomy patients to one of three groups in two hospitals to assess the effect of two preoperative instruction methods on stress and postoperative patient outcomes.

On analysis, patient outcomes were hospital dependent, rather than process dependent. While the authors had believed the two hospitals were similar (in terms of size, location, clientele, type, and financial structure), the study results led them to conclude otherwise. The investigators postulated that the statistically significant differences between groups in one hospital—on such outcomes as mean narcotic dose, stress levels, complications, and length of stay—were related to the context of patient care delivery rather than to the experimental interventions.[15]

As a result of their unexpected findings, Hegyvary and Chamings[15] strongly cautioned against simplistic cause-and-effect approaches for studying the complex situations found in healthcare. According to these authors, because of the multitude of variables in these complex systems, such methods would lead to spurious results. They recognized that combinations of variables and context are important. Without actually saying it, these investigators suggested that what matters is the relationship between things.

Evolving World-Views

Using the Newtonian approach, scientific discoveries into the early twentieth century appeared to be confirming the presence of immutable laws in the physical world. Early in the twentieth century, however, the clockwork metaphor could not be reconciled with the significant findings of scientists like Albert Einstein. According to Reed, modernist philosophies and empiricist approaches to knowledge development were failing to produce an "empirical base for ultimate meaning and truth about human beings and their world."[1] This paradigm was too narrow and limited, not only in understanding human relationships, but also in the majority of things in nature.[16]

As the mechanistic world-view of the modernist period began to lose support, the postmodern period emerged. Although postmodernism is a philosophy, it is also a social movement. Identified as a time of "paradigms lost," postmodernism heavily affected the nursing profession's approach to knowledge development.[1] The postmodern period "challenges the modernist idea of a single, transcendent meaning of reality and the importance of the search for empirical patterns that correspond to and represent ultimate meaning."[1] Postmodernism requires letting go of the premise that there is only one truth and accepting the idea that truth is based on your own reality—who you are, where you are, and what you have experienced. This dramatic revolution in thinking left many scientists feeling that "the gods have fled."[1]

Nursing's Adaptation to the Changing World-view

While those of the modernist era tended to dichotomize inquiry (research versus practice, inductive versus deductive reasoning, qualitative versus quantitative data), the shift to postmodernism engendered more complementary views of inquiry. As Rodgers noted, "the key to quality and meaningful inquiry lies with understanding the philosophical underpinnings of the method, in other words what does it 'mean' to study something a particular way."[13] The philosophical assumption that people interpret their lives based on their unique understanding to make sense of their experiences makes narratives, story, discourse, art, literature, literary analysis, and dance valuable research tools that would not have merit with a reductionistic framework of inquiry. The postmodernist approach resonated with nurses' experience, but nursing science, like all other sciences, would require some time for the revolution to occur.

Nursing's adaptation to the changing world-view is evident in the history of nursing theory development. Florence Nightingale was probably the first to recognize the importance of relationships and interactions among factors that affect health. Nightingale's understanding of the relationship between health and environment is said to have initiated the development of nursing knowledge through research and theory.[17;18] In the early 1900s, however, reductionistic beliefs reigned. This reductionistic stronghold created a century-long stall between Nightingale's understanding of the relationship of health and environment and the development of nursing theories outside of the reductionistic paradigm.

With the 1950s came the scientific revolution grounded in a systems theory paradigm. Those nurse theorists that built their frameworks on systems theory saw the whole human as a bio-psycho-social and sometimes spiritual being. These theorists viewed health as a continuum and believed the person is both separate from the environment while in interaction with it. Knowledge was sought by studying the parts. While there was recognition that the whole was greater than the sum of the parts, the belief was still firmly ingrained that one could understand the whole by studying the parts. Theorists who embraced this concept included King,[19] Orem,[20] Neuman,[21] Peplau,[21] and Roy,[22] among others.

In the 1960s, important themes which revolved around relationship and context emerged and laid the groundwork for nursing in the twenty-first century. Those themes built on an increasing understanding that the complexity of nursing required multiple theories, and that all theories need to be tested before being dismissed or modified. The methodology used for testing depends on the stage of the theory's development, and these themes established the boundaries necessary for nursing to focus and creatively expand its research efforts.[17]

The seismic shift signaling the change of nursing theory away from a reductionistic paradigm, towards a world-view of wholeness was Martha Rogers' theory: The Science of Unitary Human Beings.[23] Her work in the 1960s and 1970s influenced future theory development by refocusing nursing care on the relationship between people and their environment, focusing on the importance of pattern recognition.[24] She described people in terms of pandimensionality, taking into account the complex nature of the human being. She moved nursing beyond the bio-psycho-social concept of compartmentalized beings to addressing the whole. Rosemary Parse described the impact made by Martha Rogers' ideas as "an earthquake."[25]

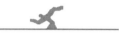

The seismic shift signaling the change of nursing theory away from a reductionistic paradigm, towards a world-view of wholeness was Martha Rogers' theory: The Science of Unitary Human Beings.

Margaret Newman[26] discussed the challenge that Rogers' theory created for the nursing discipline. While nursing researchers and theorists were grappling with the need for a scientific revolution that would move nursing away from the accepted reductionistic ways of knowing, Martha Rogers challenged the profession to step outside of its old paradigm into a world not yet imagined. Rogers recognized the need for new methodologies that transcended traditional approaches to knowledge development.[24]

The idea of human interaction with the environment introduced by Rogers[24] shifted the focus from "doing to" toward "being with." Parse describes this shift as "moving beyond the meaning moment to what is not yet."[27] Looking at this theory from a Complexity Science paradigm, one can see an emphasis on the relationship between dynamic beings, rather than on the beings themselves, in the creation of responses that cannot be reduced or measured in the reductionistic tradition.

Martha Rogers' work was the "tipping point" from the modernist to a postmodernist nursing science landscape. This reflected a shift from the Newtonian system world-view to an interactive complex world-view. Others followed Roger's lead. Margaret Newman introduced her Theory of Health as Expanding Consciousness[28;29] and Rosemary Parse offered her Human Becoming Theory.[27] These theorists recognized the interactional nature of human beings not only with each other, but also with their environments. Watson[30] took this relationship a step further, recognizing that caring is foundational in the process of belonging to other human beings in a unified, relational connectedness. Leininger[31] offered unique insights into culture care as a foundational construct that respects the diversity of all by adopting a transcultural approach to caring. The general agreement in all of these theories was that the metaparadigm of human-universe-health process was nursing's phenomenon of concern.

Wright[23] reminded us, however, that definitions of terms in this process differed according to one of two world-views. Note that the first world-view is reductionistic—it can be understood by studying the parts—and the latter is postmodern, consisting of nonlinear, unpredictable relationships between things, not the things themselves. Barrett,[32] a noted theorist and Rogerian scholar, summarily dismissed the idea that one of these world-views should be considered superior, stating that both were required to create necessary methods for inquiry and practice expansive enough for the activities of the discipline. While Barrett simply said the two paradigms were just different, a philosophic dilemma remained—how could both be true? For as Rodgers[13] noted, all human endeavors are shaped and described by philosophy. According to Rodgers, philosophy provides the means for evaluating knowledge development and for the basis for the values from which to determine knowledge development priorities and modes of inquiry.

Philosophers Kuhn and Feyarabend had swayed rationalists in the 1960s to accept that Newtonian theories and those based on relativistic mechanics are incommensurable because of the assumptions underlying each paradigm.[33] This only served to escalate the concern that nursing knowledge built on these two world-views and the theories emanating from them were violations of the "logic of truth [in particular] the principle of noncontradiction."[34] The paradox is that there is an explanation for the legitimacy of each world-view and subsequent theories.

Complexity Science provides a framework for inquiry that helps explain how the world functions, not how we wish it would function. It addresses paradoxes and sees them as points of strengths. Complexity Science promotes "both/and" rather than "either/or." It helps resolve the philosopher's concern about violating the logic of truth. The framework provided by Complexity Science creates a juxtaposition of the two world-views into a complementary arrangement rather than the either/or choice some philosophers identified as necessary. Complexity Science supports a broader world-view, recognizing that human relationships are never simple. When people are interacting, the results are inherently unpredictable and nonlinear.

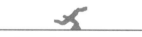

Complexity Science promotes "both/and" rather than "either/ or." It helps resolve the philosopher's concern about violating the logic of truth.

So Where Does Complexity Science Get Us?

In any discussion of nursing theory, it is essential to be mindful that care improvement through clinical application is the purpose of theory development.[2] There is growing realization that as medical care has evolved from the provision of primarily acute care to primarily chronic care, less of what we do as healthcare professionals impacts health outcomes in any predictable way. The unexpected can and does happen. Overtly recognizing this evolution in care requires new ways of thinking and acting. As Abraham Maslow was noted to say many years ago, "If the only tool you have is a hammer, you tend to see every problem as a nail." For several hundred years, our only tool has been Newton's hammer of linear problem solving.

The evidence that linear problem solving approaches are inadequate is mounting. Traditional Total Quality Management (TQM), borrowed by healthcare because of its success in industry, is a widely implemented and primarily linear problem solving approach. TQM in healthcare, however, has been shown to have nearly a seventy-five percent failure rate.[35] Instead of predictable improvements, small interventions often produce large effects, while some large interventions create very small or unintended effects. This realization is the first step in denouncing the artificial boundary imposed by an underlying assumption that the relationship between cause and effect is always linear. If we accept the idea that we can only predict and control in simple or complicated situations, where the sum of the parts is equal to the whole, then we begin to recognize that linear theories assuming an ability to predict and control are not sufficient to improve care for our patients with truly complex health problems.

There is growing realization that as medical care has evolved from the provision of primarily acute care to primarily chronic care, less of what we do as healthcare professionals impacts health outcomes in any predictable way.

Given a seventy-five percent failure rate for traditional change initiatives, one should question the validity of the underlying assumptions of our current linear theories. Prolific author and nurse researcher Janice Morse[2] would view the continued and predominant use of linear theories in healthcare delivery as an ethical concern. If we know that the linear theories are not working, we are—Morse contends—ethically bound to stop using them. Progress has been slow in resolving the inadequacy of a dominant, mechanistic world-view. A new metaphor, then, could provide an alternative lens that encompasses the simple, complicated, and complex situations in nursing care.

Paul Cilliers, a noted scholar currently studying the implications of Complexity Science for ethics, law, and justice, argues that the "technologisation of science is changing the relationship between science and philosophy in radical ways."[12] In the past, if something was too complex to understand, the analytical method supported dividing the entity into units, analyzing them, and then reassembling them. In reality, the whole is not just greater than the sum of the parts; it is different, unpredictable, and influenced by the relationship between the parts. There is growing understanding that in complex systems, the analytical mechanical approach destroys what it seeks to understand.

Ziegler identifies that the link between theory and the delivery of quality nursing care is the nurse in practice. Nursing action, then, is dependent on how the nurse uses knowledge, which is predicated on her thinking. If nurses are taught to believe in and use only linear, rational problem solving approaches, it will negatively influence every aspect of nursing, including the quality of nursing care delivered, nursing education, research designed to test theory, and the types of theory generated.[4] Furthermore, it will negatively affect how the nurse perceives their success or failure in caring for patients when the actions they take fail to deliver the intended outcomes. Nursing practice using a particular theory, then, has the capability to affect the quality of care delivered, and also the satisfaction that nurses have in their ability to provide care.

Nursing needs world-views and theories that encompass both linear and nonlinear problem solving. Susan K. Leddy, nurse educator and researcher, suggested that such theories are essential for coherence of nursing knowledge. According to Leddy, an inclusive, rather than exclusive, world-view can encourage alternate ways of thinking, creativity, and knowledge synthesis.[36] Complexity Science provides such a complementary perspective, facilitating a new way to describe, understand, and use nursing theory within boundaries appropriate to the concepts and constructs of interest in nursing. Such specificity will enable nursing science to advance beyond the linear theoretical models that can neither explain nor predict the nonlinear outcomes so prevalent in nursing.

Powers and Knapp define theory as "a set of statements that tentatively describe, explain, or predict relationships between concepts that have been systematically selected and organized as an abstract representation of some phenomenon."[37] It is, therefore, a way to describe the relationship between things. An important assumption of Newtonian science or the "received view" is that prediction and control of phenomenon is achievable, and that linear relationships exist between the concepts involved in the phenomenon. The aim of early nursing theory was to gain control over a phenomenon. A growing realization is that simple theories cannot adequately describe very complex realities.[12]

Complexity Science, developed over the last forty years, challenges the assumption that control is possible when there are complex adaptive systems involved in the phenomenon. Complexity Science provides the framework for making wise choices about the problem solving strategies to use in any given situation. Such wisdom should bring with it the confidence of knowing we have chosen our actions wisely. Rodgers admonishes nurse researchers to avoid the reductionism that inquiry seems to breed and find a way to discover the interactions among systems that affect health.[13] Palmer explains that wisdom is the richness created by using a nonlinear process to determine truth.[9]

Envisioning Nursing and Healthcare Using the Complexity Science Framework

Nursing is a complex, multi-dimensional interacting process between humans experiencing a journey in health.[38] The enactment of this process is hindered by the current context of nursing practice. With the explosion of scientific knowledge, healthcare delivery was splintered into specialties based on body systems, age groups, and sub-specializations. As a result, healthcare delivery became fragmented. Increasing use of technology promoted "doing to" rather than "caring for." According to Milton, the focus shifted toward positivistic development of biomedical and pharmaceutical interventions aimed at prolonging life and eliminating disease.

Some nurse leaders believe that current developments in nursing and healthcare in the United States have set the stage for a dramatic transformation.[39] In the ocean, estuaries exist where rivers and sea merge. In this mixture of fresh and salt water, there are organisms not found in the ocean or in fresh water. These estuaries provide a place where creative metamorphosing evokes the emergence of new life forms.[40] There is a critical need to create a metaphorical estuary that promotes such a metamorphosis and new beginnings in healthcare, a "place where the common and the uncommon can come together and emerge as a transforming force for a new way of providing healthcare."[40]

Conditions identified by Picard and Henneman that make nursing and healthcare ripe for sea change include the patient safety initiatives of the Institute of Medicine (IOM).[41] Transforming the work environment of nurses, for example, was identified as central to the transformation of patient care, and will require revolutionary, not evolutionary, changes in practice that radically alter the conversations and the way work gets done in practice environments.[39] The IOM suggested developing learning environments, using knowledge to guide practice, and fostering reflective, caring, and compassionate organizations for patients and health care professionals. In one of the early IOM publications on healthcare quality, Plsek[42] advocated using Complexity Science as a theoretical framework. Improving relationships and communication among healthcare professionals will be crucial to this transformative process.[43]

Milton[38] links improved relationships and communication to the process of knowing. In healthcare, patient information is dynamic. As patient conditions increase in complexity, information in isolation becomes less and less useful for decision making. Only when all members of the healthcare team and the patient collaboratively share their information can

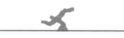

Wisdom is the richness created by using a nonlinear process to determine truth.

outcomes be optimized.[44;45] This corresponds to Capra's[46] networks and webs of relationships—of primary importance in describing reality—and is representative of the complementary and comprehensive framework provided by Complexity Science for improved clinical decision making.

Improved clinical decision making is the desired outcome of effective nursing. Among other things, good clinical decision making requires adequate time to provide care and to reflect on practice. What nursing needs is a type of estuary where technology and human interrelating meet to support effective decision making and creative metamorphosing. What does the future hold for such a vision?

According to Nash (Sue Nash in discussion with author February 9, 2007), there are places where an estuary exists to foster relational connecting and creative metamorphosing. For example, at M. D. Anderson Cancer Center on their Palliative Care Unit, healthcare professionals, families, and patients meet over tea in a living room-like setting. In this setting creative dialogue and conversations are facilitated, leading to shared understandings and improved care planning. Contrast this to the ten white coats standing over the gowned patient in a bed, with family in the background or, more commonly, at a time when the family and the nurse cannot be present.

While many healthcare professionals would likely cite time as a barrier to such an approach, there are studies that demonstrate that relational con-

necting, while it takes time, actually saves time overall and improves outcomes, especially as patient complexity increases. In one study, Baggs and
Schmitt[47] found that working together in an intensive care unit was described as working as a team, maintaining a patient-centered focus, and
sharing. Success relied on availability and receptivity to collaboration, a
place to collaborate, and competence of the participants.

Curly, McEachern, and Speroff[44] also chose a relational process of daily
patient rounds for a patient population with very complex and individualized needs, rather than implementing predetermined or routine care
paths. All involved healthcare professionals were included in rounds. In
this randomized, controlled trial, those patients in the interdisciplinary
rounds group had both significantly lower lengths of stay and lower
charges for their hospital stay. Further studies are needed, using Complexity Science as the framework for inquiry, to test the impact of improved
relational connections and the context of care on outcomes.[10]

As healthcare environments and professional practice change, supported by the Complexity Science framework for inquiry, education must
also change. Students today are typically immersed in what Palmer calls the
"mythical but dominant model of truth-knowing and truth-telling."[9] Such
is also true of nursing education.[36] This linear model assumes the expert
has knowledge and passes that knowledge to amateurs, taking care to as-
sure that only objective knowledge flows down without any interjection of
subjectivity from either the amateur or the expert. True education will require educators to be guides who take students on an "inner journey toward more truthful ways of seeing and being in the world."[9] A Complexity
Science framework could help nursing students develop and organize nursing practice knowledge in a much more coherent and complementary way.
Such a framework will require the creation of a "community of truth,"[9]
where the subject of interest is available for relationships with those who
wish to gain understanding. By entering into circular and dynamic patterns of communication where observations and interpretations are shared,
truth becomes a nonlinear process of emergence.

What then does the future hold? Rodgers[13] proposed that the future of
nursing knowledge must be created and cannot be predicted. This statement is congruent with the tenets of Complexity Science.[35] The emerging
theory of Complexity Science can help inform nursing practice, offer new
insights into the unpredictable nature of the dynamic relationship called

nursing, and assist in organizing nursing knowledge. The knowledge, once organized, can be used repeatedly in practice to guide decision making— not to predict and control. The nurse, as she enters a new situation will apply this lens to gain a gestalt of the situation.

In a study of nurse decision making, the nurse participants repeatedly described decision making processes that involved looking for the connection between things— including drug administration and patient response—and for expected patterns as well as deviations from expected patterns.[48] The decision making routines described included simultaneously looking for simple, complicated, and complex interactions and responding appropriately—representing their use of both simple and nonlinear decision making.[48] How much more quickly could nurses move from novice to expert if these skills were taught using a Complexity Science framework?

Understanding Complexity Science can assist us in creating a desired future. Change in a complex adaptive system, such as healthcare, occurs as system agents (ideas, people, nursing units, and clients) interact over time. As system agents interact, a change or transformation occurs in each entity involved in the interaction. By creating spaces or estuaries for these transforming exchanges, new structures and patterns will be created that better meet the needs of patients.[35] Assuring a context of care that truly supports transforming exchanges is critical to making the best patient care decisions.

Nursing needs a new paradigm that can exploit nursing's ways of knowing[49] and foster knowledge development for expert nursing practice. Complexity Science is emerging as the paradigm that can advance nursing theory, knowledge, and practice. Complexity Science provides us a framework for inquiry that can be used to develop nursing theories that help nurses make sense of patient care experiences and better solve problems in practice. Only by recognizing and responding appropriately to the nonlinear dynamics present in healthcare will we begin to gain a true understanding of how best to improve health outcomes and create nurturing organizations that support the clients they serve and the needs of healthcare professionals providing care.

Mary L. Gambino, PhD, RN, is assistant dean for community affairs, director of nursing continuing education, and a clinical assistant professor at the University of Kansas. She holds graduate appointments in the School of Nursing and the School of Medicine's Health Policy & Management department at Kansas University Medical Center in Kansas City, Kansas. She teaches Complexity Science at the graduate level. Her research interests cover healthcare quality improvement, collaboration, decision making, and Complexity Science. Prior to her academic career, Dr. Gambino held senior management positions in managed care organizations.

Works Cited

1. P. G. Reed, "A Treatise on Nursing Knowledge Development for the 21st Century: Beyond Postmodernism," in *Perspectives on Nursing Theory* 4th ed. (Philadelphia: Lippincott Williams & Wilkins, 2004), 561-572, 563, 562, 563.

2. J. M. Morse, "Nursing Scholarship: Sense and Sensibility," *Nursing Inquiry* 3, no. 2 (1996): 74-82.

3. "Michel de Montaigne," 2008. Available from http://plato.standford.edu/archives/win2006/entries/montaigne.

4. S. M. Ziegler, "Introduction to Theory-Directed Nursing Practice," in *Theory-Directed Nursing Practice* 2nd ed. (New York: Springer Publishing Company, 2005), 1-4.

5. T. S. Kuhn, *The Structure of Scientific Revolutions* 2nd ed. (Chicago: University of Chicago Press, 1970).

6. R. T. Pascale, M. Millemann, and L. Gioja, *Surfing the Edge of Chaos: The Laws of Nature and the New Laws of Business* (New York: Crown Publishers, 2000), 1.

7. J. T. Klein, "Interdisciplinarity and Complexity: An Evolving Relationship," *Emergence: Complexity and Organization* 6, no. 1-2 (2004): 2-10.

8. B. Zimmerman, C. Lindberg, and P. Plesk, *Insights from Complexity Science for Healthcare Leaders* (Irving: VHA Inc., 2001).

9. P. J. Palmer, *The Courage to Teach: Exploring the Inner Landscape of a Teacher's Life* (San Francisco: Jossey-Bass, 1998), 100, 6, 101.

10. R. A. Anderson et al., "Case Study Research: The View From Complexity Science," *Qualitative Health Research* 15, no. 5 (2005): 669-685.

11. M. M. Waldrop, *Complexity: The Emerging Science at the Edge of Order and Chaos* (New York: Simon & Schuster, 1992), 327-328.

12. P. Cilliers, *Complexity and Postmodernism: Understanding Complex Systems* (London: Routledge, 1998), 1.

13. B. L. Rodgers, *Developing Nursing Knowledge: Philosophical Traditions and Influences* (Philadelphia: Lippincott Williams & Wilkins, 2005), 194.

14. D. E. Johnson, "Theory in Nursing: Borrowed and Unique," *Nursing Research* 17 (1968): 206-209.

15. S. T. Hegyvary and P. A. Chamings, "The Hospital Setting and Patient Care Outcomes. Part II," *Journal of Nursing Administration* 5, no. 4 (1975): 36-42.

16. T. Petzinger, Jr., "A New Model for the Nature of Business: It's Alive! — Forget the Mechanical — Today's Leaders Embrace the Biological," *Wall Street Journal,* 1999.

17. A. I. Meleis, *Theoretical Nursing: Development & Progress* 3rd ed. (Philadelphia: Lippincott, 1997).

18. M. K. Senesac and P. M. Sato, "Imagining Nursing Practice: The Roy Adaptation Model in 2050," *Nursing Science Quarterly* 20 (2007): 47-50.

19. I. M. King, *A Theory for Nursing: Systems, Concepts, Process* (New York: John Wiley & Sons, Inc., 1981).

20. D. E. Orem, *Nursing: Concepts of Practice* 2nd ed. (New York: McGraw-Hill Book Company, 1980).

21. B. Neuman and J. Fawcett, *The Neuman Systems Model* 4th ed. (Upper Saddle River: Prentice Hall, 2002).

22. C. Roy and H. Andrews, *The Roy Adaptation Model* 2nd ed. (Stamford: Appleton & Lange, 1999).

23. B. W. Wright, "The Evolution of Rogers' Science of Unitary Human Beings: 21st Century Reflections," *Nursing Science Quarterly* 20 (2007): 64-67.

24. M. E. Rogers, *An Introduction to the Theoretical Basis of Nursing* (Philadelphia: F.A. Davis, 1970).

25. R. R. Parse, "Investing the Legacy: Martha A. Rogers' Voice Will Not Be Silenced," *Visions: The Journal of Rogerian Nursing Science* 5 (1997): 7-11, 7.

26. M. A. Newman, "Theory for Nursing Practice," *Nursing Science Quarterly* 7 (1994): 153-157.

27. R. R. Parse, "The Human Becoming Theory in Practice," in *Illuminations: The Human Becoming Theory in Practice and Research* (New York: National League for Nursing Press, 1995), 77-80, 83.

28. M. A. Newman, *A Developing Discipline: Selected Works of Margaret Newman* (New York: National League for Nursing Press, 1995).

29. M. A. Newman, *Health as Expanding Consciousness* 2nd ed. (Sudbury: Jones and Bartlett Publishers, 2000).

30. J. Watson, *Caring Science as Sacred Science* (Philadelphia: F.A. Davis Company, 2005).

31. M. M. Leininger and M. R. McFarland, *Transcultural Nursing: Concepts, Theories, Research, and Practice* 3rd ed. (New York: McGraw-Hill, Medical Publishing, 2002).

32. E. A. Barrett, "What Is Nursing Science?," *Nursing Science Quarterly* 15 (2002): 51-60.

33. W. H. Newton-Smith, *The Rationality of Science* (Boston: Routledge & Kegan Paul, 1981).

34. J. F. Kikuchi and H. Simmons, "The Whole Truth and Progress in Nursing Knowledge Development," in *Truth in Nursing Inquiry* (Thousand Oaks: Sage Publications, 1996), 5-18, 6.

35. E. E. Olson and others, *Facilitating Organization Change: Lessons from Complexity Science* (San Francisco: Jossey-Bass/Pfeiffer, 2001).

36. S. K. Leddy, "Scholarly Dialogue. Toward a Complementary Perspective on Worldviews," *Nursing Science Quarterly* 13 (2000): 225-233.

37. B. A. Powers and T. R. Knapp, *A Dictionary of Nursing Theory and Research* 2nd ed. (Thousand Oaks: Sage Publications, 1995).

38. C. L. Milton, "Information and Human Freedom: Nursing Implications and Ethical Decision-Making in the 21st Century," *Nursing Science Quarterly* 20 (2007): 33-36.

39. C. Picard and E. A. Henneman, "Theory-Guided Evidence-Based Reflective Practice: An Orientation to Education for Quality Care," *Nursing Science Quarterly* 20 (2007): 39-42.

40. S. S. Bunkers, "Sea Change in Nursing," *Nursing Science Quarterly* 20 (2007): 37-38.

41. Institute of Medicine, *Keeping Patients Safe: Transforming the Work Environment of Nurses* (Washington, D.C.: National Academies Press, 2004).

42. P. E. Plsek, "Redesigning Healthcare with Insights from the Science of Complex Adaptive Systems," in *Crossing the Quality Chasm: A New Health System for the 21st Century* (Washington, D.C.: National Academies Press, 2001), 309-322.

43. A. Suchman, "A New Theoretical Foundation for Relationship-Centered Care: Complex Responsive Processes of Relating," *Journal of General Internal Medicine* 21 (2006): 40-44.

44. C. Curly, J. McEachern, and T. Speroff, "A Firm Trial of Interdisciplinary Rounds on the Inpatient Medical Wards," *Medical Care* 36, no. Suppl (1998): AS4-12.

45. W. A. Knaus et al., "An Evaluation of Outcome From Intensive Care in Major Medical Centers," *Annals of Internal Medicine* 104 (1986): 410-418.

46. F. Capra, *The Web of Life* (New York: Anchor Books Doubleday, 1996).

47. J. G. Baggs and M. H. Schmitt, "Nurses' and Resident Physicians' Perceptions of the Process of Collaboration in an MICU," *Research in Nursing & Health* 20 (1997): 71-80.

48. M. L. Kinnaman, *Exploring the Clinical Decision-Making Strategies of Nurses*. Paper presented at Sigma Theta Tau International, 2007, at Kansas City.

49. B. A. Carper, "Fundamental Patterns of Knowing in Nursing," *Advances in Nursing Science* 1, no. 1 (1978): 13-23.

50. "Rationalism," 2008. Available from http://www.merriam-webster.com/dictionary/rationalism.

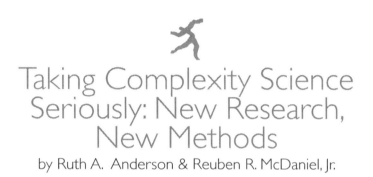

Taking Complexity Science Seriously: New Research, New Methods

by Ruth A. Anderson & Reuben R. McDaniel, Jr.

...organization and structures do not have to be hierarchical and top-down, but instead could be emergent forms that result from 'bottom up' processes of interaction.[1]

When we think our organizations are machines, the problem is to get the parts to fit right and keep them oiled. We now understand that healthcare organizations are not machines but rather complex adaptive systems. Therefore, we do not have as our managerial objective simply getting the parts right and oiling them.

Opening Thoughts:
A Grounding in Complex Adaptive Systems

Complex adaptive systems (CASs) are made up of agents, like nurses and patients, that learn and that relate to each other and to the environment in nonlinear ways. A key result of this pattern of interaction is self-organization. Complex adaptive systems organize themselves in fairly stable patterns of relationships that are not governed by hierarchical intent. Such a pattern could be how nursing assistants, nurses, and nurse managers interact in a nursing home. Emergent properties are a second result of these interactions. Emergent properties are characteristics of the system—like the well-being of patients or infection rates—that cannot be completely understood by knowing the characteristics of the system's parts. The third result of nonlinear interaction among agents is co-evolution. CASs evolve in response to environmental conditions, Complexity Science influenced our research group and our research has influenced how Complexity Science is understood in healthcare; our research group interacted with staff in nursing homes and we were both affected. Nonlinearity, coupled with feed-forward feedback information, leads to fundamental uncertainty, so CASs are full of surprises.[2;3]

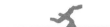

Because we now understand that healthcare organizations are complex adaptive systems, we also understand that our strategies for learning about them must be different than when we believed we could learn about them as if they were machines.

Because we now understand that healthcare organizations are complex adaptive systems, we also understand that our strategies for learning about them must be different than when we believed we could learn about them as if they were machines.[4-6] These strategies must acknowledge that the relationships among clinical professionals and the quality of those relationships indeed may be more important than the quality of the professionals themselves.[7] We need to understand that healthcare quality is an emergent property of the system and not something that that can be imposed successfully from the outside.[1;8] We must recognize that uncertainty is often the result of system characteristics, not merely a lack of information.[2-4;6;8-10] As we have come face-to-face with these new insights, we have had to develop new models for our research studies, invent new research methods, and learn new ways to use old methods.

Our understanding of Complexity Science caused us to study very closely the everyday, micro-interactions in nursing homes, the focus of our organizational research. For example, we examined the question of how a nursing assistant and nurse talk about a particular patient. It also caused us to appreciate that our research and interactions in a nursing home affected what is happening in the nursing home as well as our research. Realization of the co-evolutionary process caused us to extend our understanding of research and seek to provide feedback to the nursing home through such strategies as training and exit consultation.[11] These steps, not previously part of our research routines and interactions, generated new insights in our research.

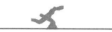

Self-organization is a property of all social systems that operates whether we recognize it or not. By recognizing it, however, managers can begin to influence it to facilitate better outcomes.

The purpose of this chapter is to share how Complex Adaptive Systems Theory has shaped our research program. We present a research model for healthcare organizations which we developed from our understandings of complex adaptive systems. We created this model to enable us to study healthcare organizations in more meaningful ways. We then share an overview of a program of research we conducted using this model as a guide. We identify and describe a number of peer-reviewed published papers that grew out of this research, as well as meaningful insights about the process of research itself.

The Complexity-Inspired Research Model

This research model stemmed from our interest in relationships among management practices, the nature of staff interactions, and quality of care in nursing homes.[12] The conceptual model illustrated in Figure 1 has been the basis for a series of research studies. Developing the model, derived from Complexity Science theories of CASs,[13] was a necessary step in going from the broader complexity theory to manageable research questions and hypotheses. The section will describe "how this was done" and give examples of what was done.

The model is grounded in our understanding of self-organization and factors which affect this process. Anderson, Issel, and McDaniel[12] reflected on the importance and universality of self-organization:

Self-organization is a property of all social systems that operates whether we recognize it or not. By recognizing it,
however, managers can begin to influence it to facilitate
better outcomes. Self-organizing is the process by which
people mutually adjust their behaviors in ways needed to
cope with changing internal and external environmental
demands.[12]

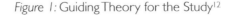

Figure 1: Guiding Theory for the Study[12]

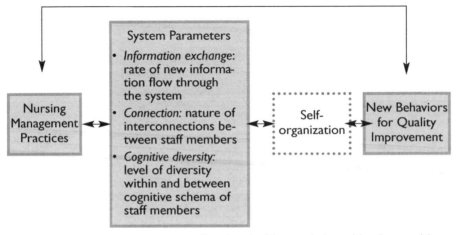

Reprinted with permission with minor revisions.

Three factors, or system parameters as they are called in Complexity
Science, which have a strong influence on self-organization are: the rate of
new information flow through the system; the nature of connections
among people; and diversity of cognitive schema.[13] The following definitions build on Stacey's[13] conceptualizations of these system parameters:

- *Rate of new information flow.* Of particular importance to self-organization is new information flow created by social interaction. When
  interacting people exchange new information, they generate new understandings and, thus, new knowledge.[14] With this knowledge, people learn, their behaviors change,[15] and they are capable of something
  new.[16;17] Thus, effective management practices would be ones that
  foster new information flow.

- *Number and nature of connections.* Networks develop when staff interact regularly to complete work.[18] Because of this network of connections, local changes in behavior can give rise to system-wide change.[19] Thus, effective management practices would be ones that foster a greater number, variety, and quality of connections among people[20-23] in the nursing home, thus influencing a capacity for new behaviors.

- *Diversity of cognitive schema.* Cognitive schemas are the mental models by which people understand and make sense of information.[24] Diverse schemas arise from education, social or cultural backgrounds, roles in the organization, age cohorts,[25] and external collaboration.[26] Effective management practices would be ones that seek diverse opinions in problem solving.[27] Sensemaking that considers multiple perspectives (registered nurses, nurse assistants, medical doctors, and social workers), for example, leads to rich interpretation of a nursing home resident situation and suggests what actions are most appropriate.[28]

In this model, we have used these system parameters and the concept of self-organization to understand and examine how nursing management practices (NMPs) are associated with better resident outcomes in nursing homes.[12;29-31] System parameters foster conditions that:

- allow people to create and recreate meaning of events;

- provide opportunities for higher-order learning that changes beliefs as opposed to simply knowing facts or rules;

- stimulate creativity;

- provide positive feedback (feedback that moves a system away from status quo); and

- offer opportunities for reflection and evaluation of performance.[4;13]

NMPs can both positively and negatively impact system parameters and self-organizing processes, thus explaining why certain NMPs are associated with better resident outcomes. Supported by appropriate relationship patterns and NMPs, self-organization allows people to develop new behaviors needed to cope with internal and external demands while supporting high-quality care. For example, by "pitching-in," a charge nurse can connect (*connection*) with a frustrated nursing assistant (NA) who is caring for a resident who is displaying early warning signs of acute illness. While pitching-in (*connection*), the nurse can "listen" to the NA and hear that the resident "doesn't look right" (*information exchange*). The nurse can immediately assess and interpret resident symptoms, interact with the NA to generate new information (*cognitive diversity*), and together develop more appropriate strategies for intervening to prevent the acute illness. Because the nurse pitched-in, she now has an open door to "give feedback"

Table 1: Program of empirical research; themes and topics

Complexity view of participation in decision making
- RN participation in decision making and improvement in patient outcomes[30]
- RN and MD participation in decision making and hospital ownership conversion[52]
- Informal versus formal participation in decision making and nurse influence over final choices[34;61]

Complexity view of nursing management practices
- Relationship-oriented management practices (participation in decision making, leadership, communication, less rule enforcement) and patient outcomes[12]
- Availability of clinical professionals and patient outcomes[33]
- Availability of clinical professionals and staff turnover[32]
- Administrative climate, communication patterns, and staff turnover[36]
- "Paying attention" as a management practice to protect patients from harm[48]
- "The Golden Rule" as a common management practice with potentially suboptimal results for patients[44]

Complexity view of relationships
- Typical relationship patterns as facilitators and barriers to patient care[45]
- Complexity view of case studies as a method for studying relationship patterns and whole systems[28]
- Relationship as a basis for effective sensemaking[45]
- Nurse and physician patterns of communication and impact on quality of care processes[39]
- Relationship between nurses, other staff, and the system as a basis for quality of care processes[31]
- Connections among staff and staff diversity for innovation in care planning; effect of differing interpretation of regulations[11]
- Relationships between staff and family and impact on care quality and staff well-being[40]
- Connecting nursing home participants to the researchers and research results; opportunities for improving practices[11]

(*cognitive diversity*) to the NA and to "coach" and "praise" (*cognitive diversity*) her as she implements nursing interventions. On the other hand and as commonly observed, the charge nurse could avoid the NA who is in need of help and the potential to avert the impending illness would be lost.

Themes Explored

This complexity-based research model has been used to explore NMPs in nursing homes and patterns of relationships among staff in nursing homes and their association with patient outcomes. We have been pursuing this stream of research for more than ten years and have explored a number of topics, some of which are displayed in Table 1.

Our earliest research set our current research course. The purpose of two early studies was to examine relationships between NMPs (participation in decision making; administrative climate; communication openness, accuracy and timeliness; leadership behaviors), resident outcomes, and staff turnover. Both studies used large-scale correlational survey methods. We matched the survey data to data from Medicaid Cost Reports (including variables such as nursing home size, ownership, staffing) and Minimum Data Set (MDS) information, including variables such as prevalence of infections, decubitus, and fractures. In the first study, which involved 190 nursing homes, we found that facilities with the most improvement in resident outcomes over six months had greater RN participation in decision making and no significant differences in cost.[30] This study suggested that improvements in resident outcomes depended in part on RN participation in decision making and provided empirical support for part of the research model. Specifically, participation in decision making–a management practice that alters system parameters by increasing information exchange, numbers of connections among staff, and cognitive diversity in problem solving–accounted for improvements in resident outcomes.

In the second study of over 3,000 nursing home administrators, directors of nursing, registered nurses (RNs), license practical nurses (LPNs), and nursing assistants (NAs) in 164 nursing homes, we found:

- More RN staffing predicted lower staff turnover[32] and better resident outcomes,[33;34] suggesting that better outcomes occurred when more clinical leaders were available to interact (connection) with staff (cognitive diversity).

• Nursing homes had better resident outcomes when RNs and NAs agreed on the level of NA participation in decision making (information exchange and connection), suggesting that staff interaction is necessary for improving outcomes.[35]

• Greater communication openness (connection), relationship-oriented leadership (connection), and RN participation in organizational decision making (information flow and cognitive diversity), and less reliance on rules (cognitive diversity) resulted in better resident outcomes.[12]

• Lower nursing staff turnover was related to greater communication openness (connection) and accuracy (information exchange) only when the administrative climate had clear work goals (information flow) and a merit-based reward system (connection).[36]

Overall, these results supported the hypothesis that NMPs which increased information flow, connection, and cognitive diversity improved resident outcomes.

Going On: The Current Research Course

These earlier quantitative studies gave direction, but they provided little insight into how NMPs actually worked day-to-day in nursing homes, making recommendations about their use difficult. What we needed next was a fine-grained understanding of specific NMPs that facilitated information exchange, connection, and cognitive diversity; the type of knowledge needed in order to develop feasible and culturally relevant interventions. We thus embarked on a course of research to describe and explain how relationship patterns and NMPs lead to behaviors that result in high or low quality outcomes. We sought to develop new insights into how NMPs are applied in practice, thus extending knowledge about how to use them effectively. The aims of this mixed-method case study research were to:

• describe relationship patterns;

- explore staff's and managers' understandings of relationship patterns and NMPs in use;

- compare relationship patterns and NMPs between homes with high-quality and poor-quality resident outcomes; and

- develop a model of relationship patterns and NMPs that foster better outcomes.

We conducted eight in-depth case studies ranging from four to six months in length. We collected data through observations (of meetings, staff engaged in care routines, and change of shift reports), shadowing of staff during their work day; in-depth interviews with staff from all departments and job levels (nursing, dietary, housekeeping, maintenance), and review of nursing home records (mission statements, marketing materials, handbooks). We also conducted structured interviews with nursing home residents using the Resident Experience and Assessment of Quality of Life (REAL) tool.[37] Eight nursing homes were enrolled and data was collected from over 600 residents and 770 staff members from all disciplines. Our sample of staff was racially diverse with about fifty percent being non-white.

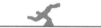

Overall, these results supported the hypothesis that NMPs which increased information flow, connection, and cognitive diversity improved resident outcomes.

Our research team itself was diverse with nursing, medicine, social work, sociology, organizational development, and management being represented. The full interdisciplinary research team participated in analysis of the data. All members read all data, including field notes of observations, and transcribed interviews. Qualitative data were coded by at least two team members using open coding to identify staff descriptions, consequences, and explanations of relationship patterns and NMPs. Coded data, with constant return to the data in context, were then analyzed to identify higher-order themes and stories in relation to quality of care. To further ensure rigor and validity, we triangulated multiple data types, used multiple data collectors and analyzers, engaged external research consultants, and obtained member checks, a strategy of asking the actual participants to assess the accuracy of the interpretations and conclusions drawn from the data. Member checks were done as part of our exit consultation process, which is described elsewhere.[11]

We began this case study with the commonly held belief that important NMPs were the exclusive purview of managers and administrators. It became evident early in the study that all levels of staff–administrators to frontline NAs–engaged in NMPs were essential to a nursing home's capacity to provide resident care. These capacity-building NMPs became the focus of our preliminary analyses. We found that NMPs were intimately interwoven with relationship patterns. Below we describe the observed relationship patterns and NMPs, and the ways in which they either facilitated or hindered good care.

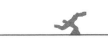

We began this case study with the belief that important NMPs were the exclusive purview of managers and administrators. It became evident that all levels of staff engaged in NMPs were essential to a nursing home's capacity to provide resident care.

Relationship patterns between discipline specific groups (NAs, LPNs, RNs, care team, managers), which were thin in most nursing homes, strongly influenced information flow.[38] When information flow was funneled through a vertical chain of command, direct care staff was excluded and information exchange and cognitive diversity in clinical problem solving were limited.[39] In another pattern, ignoring the chain of command led to rapid problem solving among a few providers, but because groups were not well connected, RN expertise was missing from decision.[39]

Four distinct patterns of care planning were found to be influenced by connection among staff. High-quality, resident-specific care planning that reached the bedside required rich relationships among staff in a variety of clinical and frontline roles. Patterns of staff and family interactions also differed. We found staff avoidance of families (run for the stairs!) was a common way staff managed relationships with demanding families, but only led to festering frustration for families and staff alike. A few nurses said that approaching families (going out of the way to say hello and ask if things are going well) was an effective way to manage relationships with families, meanwhile gathering information that might improve resident care.[40]

Relationship patterns developed by MDS nurses (nurses hired to manage resident assessments for reimbursement) differed between nursing homes. For example in one nursing home, the MDS nurses were extraordinarily connected to frontline staff and used frequent, consistent interactions to facilitate more accurate assessment and individualized care planning. Because of their network of relationships, these MDS nurses were able to describe important system issues to managers and thus stimulate system changes. In another nursing home, the MDS nurses had only a few, weak connections and thus had little knowledge with which to impact care quality; this made them feel frustrated and powerless and represented an incredible loss of potential for this nursing home.[31]

We observed that the NMP of "pitching-in" effectively created connections among staff, broke down status barriers, and facilitated teamwork.

These analyses demonstrated that it was possible for individuals to influence care in important ways by maintaining relationships across roles and disciplines. NMPs that facilitated information flow included behaviors such as listening, giving and receiving information, explaining and verifying understandings, and providing feedback. These were repeatedly described as essential NMPs.

Although connection among staff was found to be essential to high-quality care, we found it was difficult to achieve consistently. Often supervisors and floor nurses interacted with staff only to correct them; staff explained this made them feel unappreciated and unvalued.[38] Staff at all levels described the NMPs of "show appreciation," "give respect," "say thank you," and "give praise" as rare, but important for increasing staff's feelings of being appreciated and respected.[41]

Surprisingly, these NMPs do not depend on large institutional reward programs; rather, they are executed locally by individuals. We view these as capacity-building NMPs that are essential to building and maintaining connections among staff.

Related to connection, teamwork was described by staff in each nursing home as an important but elusive goal. The case study nursing homes were fraught with clique and "status" barriers between levels of staff.[38]

We observed that the NMP of "pitching-in" effectively created connections among staff, broke down status barriers, and facilitated teamwork. Managers and nurses did not need to pitch-in very often, but often enough that others perceived them as willing to pitch-in. When managers pitched-in, it validated the importance of the staff's work and provided opportunities for listening, sharing information, and giving feedback. Pitching-in usually occurred during chance encounters as managers moved through the work environment. Thus, it is a low-cost, high-benefit strategy that was used and valued by all levels of nursing home staff. Universally, pitching-in was viewed as an essential NMP by both staff and managers.[42]

The results support targeting local interaction as a powerful way to improve quality.

Lack of connection between clinical staff and NAs meant that there was little cognitive diversity in problem solving, leading to suboptimal resident outcomes.[31;39;43;44] For example, we found that CNAs made accurate observations of resident symptoms but often interpreted them inappropriately, leading to potentially poor care. This was particularly problematic, given a lack of meaningful interactions with RNs and other clinicians who could influence CNAs' interpretations of information, a process known as sensemaking. Thus, important observations made by CNAs many times never reached the clinical professionals who could have incorporated this information into resident care.[38] We found isolated examples that showed that when clinical professionals engaged in sensemaking with CNAs, interpretations were reframed and learning occurred.[31;38] Thus, sensemaking is a capacity-building NMP.

Also related to cognitive diversity is "paying attention." It involves sensitivity to surroundings, accepting nothing as routine, and encouraging staff to detect early warning signs.[45-47] While the research data contained many examples of not paying attention, they also contained powerful positive examples from staff in every position. They ranged from noticing that a resident was chilled to signs of impending stroke. Paying attention included asking questions and being persistent to ensure action was taken.[48] Paying attention is needed for early detection of signs of acute illness or other problems and, as such, is a capacity-building NMP.

We analyzed the data to describe leadership behaviors demonstrated by RNs and LPNs in administrative positions, and determined their relationship to quality of care, staff morale, and turnover. We defined leadership as engaging in behaviors that enhanced information exchange, fostered high-quality relationships (connection), and encouraged multiple perspectives in problem solving (cognitive diversity). We found a surprising lack of leadership in directors of nursing positions. However, floor nurses (usually LPNs) exemplified many of these behaviors and provided leadership at the unit level.[42] This is an example of staff engaging in NMPs in unexpected ways and suggests these behaviors will facilitate leadership throughout the organization.

Major Findings

Based on the case study data, we have developed a grounded model of local interaction among staff and emergent, global properties of the system such as work environment and quality of resident care. The model (Figure 2), based on the Complexity Science thesis that quality emerges through local

Figure 2: Grounded model of capacity building nursing management practices

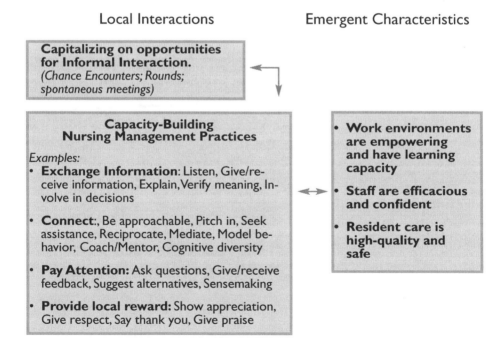

Local Interactions   Emergent Characteristics

Capitalizing on opportunities for Informal Interaction.
(Chance Encounters; Rounds; spontaneous meetings)

Capacity-Building Nursing Management Practices
Examples:
- **Exchange Information**: Listen, Give/receive information, Explain, Verify meaning, Involve in decisions

- **Connect:**, Be approachable, Pitch in, Seek assistance, Reciprocate, Mediate, Model behavior, Coach/Mentor, Cognitive diversity

- **Pay Attention:** Ask questions, Give/receive feedback, Suggest alternatives, Sensemaking

- **Provide local reward:** Show appreciation, Give respect, Say thank you, Give praise

- **Work environments are empowering and have learning capacity**

- **Staff are efficacious and confident**

- **Resident care is high-quality and safe**

interactions, describes NMPs that facilitate new information flow, connection, and cognitive diversity.[49] The results support targeting local interaction as a powerful way to improve quality. In positive local interaction patterns, people engage in effective new information exchange, develop high-quality relationships, and foster cognitive diversity in problem solving. With these patterns, staff feels respected and efficacious, and care is more resident-focused. This demonstrates the potential for nursing homes to truly improve by nurturing this hidden capacity in staff.[49]

From our time in these nursing homes, we believe that much can be done to improve care using existing nursing home staff and resources, with an intervention to improve local interaction.

The findings show that nursing homes possess a capacity for better care that is currently untapped because of poor information flow, thin connections among staff, and little cognitive diversity in care planning and problem solving. It is very exciting to see, however, that capacity-building management practices are possible and perhaps will change the face of nursing home care if practiced often and systematically.

Looking Ahead: Future Research Course

From our time in these nursing homes, we believe that much can be done to improve care using existing nursing home staff and resources, with an intervention to improve local interaction. Using the grounded model (Figure 2), we developed an intervention designed to release the capacity to improve, which is so often trapped in the local relationship patterns in nursing homes. We are testing the intervention using learning methods that have been designed specifically to be culturally relevant and accessible to staff of various levels of literacy.

We are still analyzing the case study data and have much more to learn about management practices from our data. To date, we have focused on NMPs that foster local interaction. We now are turning out attention to other NMPs. For example, we are exploring the data to compare the NMPs described by nursing home managers and staff against Weick and Sutcliffe's definition of mindfulness[50] and are developing a model of mindful management practices.[51] Other future directions will be to engage in studies of self-organization and emergence. While our work hints at self-organization, we have yet to fully understand this powerful property of complex adaptive systems (represented in dotted lines in Figure 1 because we could not observe it directly in our studies to date). We are also interested in studying quality as an emergent property in healthcare systems.

The research we reported here was primarily conducted in nursing homes. Complexity Science, however, is the anchor of many studies we have conducted in a wide variety of healthcare settings. A full accounting of these requires much more space than we have here. We point to a representative sample of studies conducted in settings other than nursing homes to provide readers with insights into the breadth of healthcare settings where these ideas are important and may be applied.

We have explored general theoretical issues in the organization and management of healthcare organizations using Complexity Science. We have shown how general management issues should be approached from a Complexity Science perspective.[4] Healthcare institutional responses to merger[52] and preparations for a bioterrorism future have been explicated[53] and special attention has been given to the notion of surprises in healthcare.[3]

McDaniel has been involved in an active program of research investigating participation in strategic decision making in hospitals. Participation has been recognized as a complicating mechanism[54] and as a strategy for increasing connections.[55] Because Complexity Science suggests a relationship between participation and performance we have looked at participation as a response to complexity[55] and examined how participation of clinical professionals and middle managers (cognitive diversity) has different effects on performance.[56]

McDaniel has also participated in an extensive program of research in primary care settings using Complexity Science as a guiding theoretical framework. Included in this work has been a careful examination of the role of relationships[57] and the role of reflection[58] in improving practice performance. A change model has been developed for quality improvement in primary care practices.[59] In an examination of change interventions in primary care it was noted that those employing principles of Complexity Science were more effective than those that did not.[60]

Organizations that deliver healthcare certainly differ from each other, but they are also very much the same. They perform critical services in ambiguous circumstances. They use a wide range of technologies. They have uncertain outcomes. And, most clearly, all of them are complex adaptive systems. Our research, done across a wide range of settings, shows that Complexity Science can help us understand the phenomenon of concern and help us to develop strategies for better organization and management of these systems.

Our Research Team Model

The "we" in this discussion of prior and future work represents creative and dedicated people who have been involved in this project over the last five years. While Anderson and McDaniel have been the anchors, everyone on the project has been a leader at some point during this project. We could write a whole chapter describing our work processes, which we designed with the intention of maximizing information exchange, connection among teammates, and cognitive diversity (no surprises there). Roles of team members varied with tasks and over time. We all engaged in data collection and we all engaged in analysis and dissemination. The team generated ideas for papers in collaboration and then one member volunteered to take the lead on analysis and initial drafts of papers. The person who assumed leadership was always listed as first author and sometimes there was a secondary lead author. Anderson was always listed last author as the study principal investigator, except in instances where she was lead author and then McDaniel was listed last (in most cases), being senior faculty. The order of authors in the middle was generally alphabetical with alternating forward and reverse order. To fully acknowledge our dear colleagues, we will list each here:

- *Natalie Ammarell, PhD*, research associate, served as project director and lead field researcher. She is largely responsible for the 100 percent retention rate for our participating nursing homes. She has a real talent for blending in during administrative staff activities and was able to provide important data about upper and mid-level management in our case nursing homes.

- *Donald (Chip) Bailey, RN, PhD,* co-investigator, brought extensive knowledge about care of older people to the project. He teaches the gerontology course at Duke University and, in 2004, his course was voted the best stand-alone gerontological nursing course in the country by the American Association of Colleges of Nursing.

- *Cathleen Colón-Emeric, MD, MHSc,* co-investigator, is a geriatrician in the Department of Medicine, Division of Geriatrics in Duke's School of Medicine and is a staff physician at Croasdaile Village Retirement Community. She is a health services researcher and has extensive experience in quality improvement related to fall and fracture prevention. In this research, she helped us to always stay close to resident care issues and care processes.

- *Kirsten Corazzini, PhD,* co-investigator, is a social gerontologist who, following her doctoral education, became a NA and worked in a nursing home to learn about care delivery first hand. In our research, she helped us to carefully explore front-line care management practices.

- *Deborah Lekan, RN, MSN,* served as a field researcher. She is a gerontological nurse clinical specialist with extensive experience in nursing homes. She worked as a nurse aide and in a variety of nursing roles (staff development coordinator, restorative care nurse, staff nurse). Because she understands clinical issues so well, in our research she provided excellent data on care team interactions.

- *Melissa Lillie MSW, LCSW,* is a licensed clinical social worker and served as a field researcher on the project. In this research, she developed great skill in participant observation of the front-line staff which provided us with great data about how staff communicated and managed their work.

- *Eleanor McConnell, RN, PhD,* co-investigator, is a nurse researcher and gerontological nurse clinical specialist. She served as a consultant to our research team on issues surrounding recruiting nursing homes into the study.

- *Mary Lynn Piven, RN, PhD* was a post-doctoral fellow in the Duke Center for Aging and Human Development (NIA AG000-29, Cohen,

PI). She specializes in mental health issues in the elderly. In addition, she helped us to explore the impact of nurses in the specialized role of Minimum Data Set (MDS) coordinator.

* *Queen Utley-Smith, RN, EdD*, co-investigator, previously worked as a nurse practitioner caring for older adults and later specialized in healthcare workforce issues. In this research, she helped us to explore how nursing home staff members manage their relationships with nursing home residents' families.

Acknowledgements:

The research team members had several sources of funding in addition to the primary study, "Outcomes of Nursing Management Practice in Nursing Homes," which was funded by the National Institute of Nursing Research (NIH 2 R01 NR003178-04A2, Anderson PI) with support of Duke's Trajectories of Aging and Care Center (NINR/NIH 2P20NR07795-04, Clipp PI). Support for Utley-Smith was provided by a minority supplement to the R01 (NINR/NIH 3 R01 NR03178-05S1, Anderson, PI). Partial support for Piven was provided by the National Institute of Aging grant AG000-29 to the Duke University Center for Aging and Human Development (Cohen, PI) and for Bailey by a John A. Hartford Foundation BAGNC Scholar grant. Colón-Emeric was supported in part by the Hartford Interdisciplinary Geriatric Research Center at Duke University (RAND/John A. Hartford Foundation 2001-0349 (Clipp, PI); RAND Project HE546, Colon-Emeric PI).

Ruth A. Anderson, PhD, RN, FAAN, is professor and chair of the PhD Program in Nursing at Duke University School of Nursing and a Senior Fellow, Duke Center for the Study of Aging and Human Development. In her research, she uses models of complex adaptive systems to study management practices in healthcare organizations. The National Institute of Health, American Nurses Foundation, and The Robert Wood Johnson Foundation have funded her research. She publishes frequently in gerontology, nursing, and healthcare management journals. Dr. Anderson is a member of the Science Advisory Board of Plexus Institute.

Reuben R. McDaniel, Jr., EdD, is professor of Information Management and holds the Charles and Elizabeth Prothro Regents Chair in Health Care Management in the McCombs School of Business at The University of Texas at Austin. He teaches courses in managing complexity and information and in knowledge management. His research interest is in management of health care organizations as complex adaptive systems. He has published in The Academy of Management Journal, Management Science, Organizational Behavior and Human Decision Processes, Gerontologist, and the Journal of Family Practice, Health Care Management Review, and Health Services Research. Dr. McDaniel is on the Science Advisory Board of Plexus Institute.

Works Cited

1. P. M. Allen, "Editorial," *Emergence: Complexity and Organization* 8, no. 1 (2006): iv-v, iv.

2. B. F. Crabtree, "Primary Care Practices Are Full of Surprises?," *Management Review* 28, no. 3 (2003): 279-283.

3. R. R. McDaniel, M. E. Jordon, and B. F. Fleeman, "Surprise, Surprise, Surprise! A Complexity View of the Unexpected," *Healthcare Management Review* 28, no. 3 (2003): 266-278.

4. R. R. McDaniel and D. J. Driebe, "Complexity Science and Health Care Management," in *Advances in Health Care Management,* ed. J. D. Blair, M. D. Fottler, and G. T. Savage., vol. 2 (Stamford: JAI press, 2001), 11-36, 26.

5. W. L. Miller et al., "Practice Jazz: Understanding Variation in Family Practices Using Complexity Science," *The Journal of Family Practice* 50, no. 10 (2001): 872-878.

6. B. Zimmerman, C. Lindberg, and P. Plsek, *Edgeware: Insights from Complexity Science for Health Care Leaders* (Irving: VHA Inc., 2001).

7. R. A. Anderson and R. R. McDaniel, "Managing Healthcare Organizations: Where Professionalism Meets Complexity Science," *Healthcare Management Review* 25, no. 1 (2000): 83-92.

8. Institute of Medicine and Committee on Quality of Healthcare in America, *Crossing the Quality Chasm: A New Healthcare System for the 21st Century* (Washington D.C.: National Academies Press, 2001).

9. P. E. Plsek and T. Greenhalgh, "Complexity Science: The Challenge of Complexity in Health Care," *BMJ* 323, no. 7313 (2001): 625-628.

10. P. E. Plsek and T. Wilson, "Complexity Science: Complexity, Leadership, and Management in Healthcare Organisations," *BMJ* 323, no. 7315 (2001): 746-749.

11. Q. Utley-Smith et al., "Exit Interview-Consultation for Research Validation and Dissemination," *Western Journal of Nursing Research* 28, no. 8 (2006): 955-973.

12. R. A. Anderson, L. M. Issel, and R. R. McDaniel, "Nursing Homes As Complex Adaptive Systems: Relationship Between Management Practice and Resident Outcomes," *Nursing Research* 52, no. 1 (2003): 12-21, 13.

13. R. Stacey, *Complexity and Creativity in Organizations* (San Francisco: Berrett-Kohler Publishers, 1996).

14. K. E. Weick and K. H. Roberts, "Collective Mind in Organizations: Heedful Interrelating on Flight Decks," *Administrative Science Quarterly* 38, no. 3 (1993): 357-381.

15. G. P. West and G. D. Meyer, "Communicated Knowledge As a Learning Foundation," *The International Journal of Organizational Analysis* 5, no. 1 (1997): 25-28.

16. A. L. Tucker, "An Empircal Study of System Improvement by Frontline Employees in Hospital Units," *Manufacturing Service Operations Management* 9, no. 4 (2007): 492-505.

17. A. C. Edmondson et al., "Learning How and Learning What: Effects of Tacit and Codified Knowledge on Performance Improvement Following Technology Adoption," *Decision Sciences* 34, no. 2 (2003): 197-223.

18. W. B. Arthur, S. N. Durlauf, and D. A. Lane, *The Economy as an Evolving Complex System II* (Reading: Addison-Wesley, 1997).

19. F. Capra, *The Web of Life* (New York: Anchor Books Doubleday, 1996).

20. A. C. Edmondson, "Psychological Safety and Learning Behavior in Work Teams," *Administrative Science Quarterly* 44, no. 2 (1999): 350-383.

21. A. C. Edmondson, "The Local and Variegated Nature of Learning in Organizations: A Group-Level Perspective," *Organization Science* 13, no. 2 (2002): 128-146.

22. I. M. Nembhard and A. C. Edmondson, "Making It Safe: The Effects of Leader Inclusiveness and Professional Status on Psychological Safety and Improvement Efforts in Health Care Teams," *Journal of Organizational Behavior* 27, no. 7 (2006): 941.

23. A. L. Tucker, I. M. Nembhard, and A. C. Edmondson, "Implementing New Practices: An Empirical Study of Organizational Learning in Hospital Intensive Care Units," *Management Science* 53, no. 6 (2007): 894-907.

24. K. E. Weick, *Sensemaking in Organizations* (Thousand Oaks: Sage, 1995).

25. N. Mark, "Beyond Individual Differences: Social Differentiation From First Principles," *American Sociological Review* 63 (1998): 309-330.

26. G. Bravo et al., "Correlates of Care Quality in Long-Term Care Facilities: A Multilevel Analysis," *Journals of Gerontology Series B-Psychological Sciences & Social Sciences* 54, no. 3 (1999): 180-188.

27. A. C. Edmondson, R. M. Bohmer, and G. P. Pisano, "Disrupted Routines: Team Learning and New Technology Implementation in Hospitals," *Administrative Science Quarterly* 46, no. 4 (2001): 685-716.

28. R. A. Anderson et al., "The Power of Relationship for High-Quality Long-Term Care," *Journal of Nursing Care Quality* 20, no. 2 (2005): 103-106.

29. C. S. Colón-Emeric et al., "Connection, Regulation, and Care Plan Innovation: A Case Study of Four Nursing Homes," *Healthcare Management Review* 31, no. 4 (2006): 337-346.

30. R. A. Anderson and R. R. McDaniel Jr., "RN Participation in Organizational Decision Making and Improvements in Resident Outcomes," *Healthcare Management Review* 24, no. 1 (1999): 7-16.

31. M. L. Piven et al., "MDS Coordinator Relationships and Nursing Home Care Processes," *Western Journal of Nursing Research* 28, no. 3 (2006): 294-309.

32. R. A. Anderson, L. M. Issel, and R. R. McDaniel, "Nursing Staff Turnover in Nursing Homes: A New Look," *Public Administration Quarterly* 21, no. 1 (1997): 69-95.

33. R. A. Anderson, P. C. Hsieh, and H. F. Su, "Resource Allocation and Resident Outcomes in Nursing Homes: Comparisons Between the Best and Worst," *Research in Nursing & Health* 21, no. 4 (1998): 297-313.

34. R. A. Anderson and R. R. McDaniel Jr., "Intensity of Registered Nurse Participation in Nursing Home Decision Making," *Gerontologist* 38, no. 1 (1998): 90-100.

35. K. Corazzini-Gomez, R. Anderson, and R. McDaniel, "Quality of Care and Nurse Aide Participation in Decision-Making About Resident Care," *Gerontologist* 42 (2002): 74.

36. R. A. Anderson, K. N. Corazzini, and R. R. McDaniel Jr., "Complexity Science and the Dynamics of Climate and Communication: Reducing Nursing Home Turnover," *Gerontologist* 44, no. 3 (2004): 378-388.

37. G. C. Uman et al., "Exit Interview-Consultation for Research Validation and Dissemination," in *Satisfaction Surveys in Long-Term Care*, ed. J. Cohen-Mansfield, F. K. Ejaz, and P. Werner. (New York: Springer Publishing Company, 2000), 166-186.

38. R. A. Anderson et al., "Nurse Assistant Mental Models, Sense Making, Care Actions and Consequences for Nursing Home Residents," *Qualitative Health Research* 15, no. 8 (2005): 1006-1021.

39. C. Colón-Emeric et al., "Patterns of Medical and Nursing Staff Communication in Nursing Homes: Implications and Insights From Complexity Science," *Qualitative Health Research* 16, no. 2 (2006): 173-188.

40. Q. Utley-Smith et al., "Staff Perceptions of Staff - Family Interactions in Nursing Homes," *Journal of Aging Studies* 23, no. 3 (2008).

41. R. A. Anderson et al., "Outcomes of Rule-Based Approaches to Management of Nursing Homes," *The Gerontologist* 64, no. Special Issue 1 (2004): 624.

42. D. Bailey et al., "Nurses: Sparks of Leadership," *The Gerontologist* 44, no. Special Issue 1 (2004): 383-384.

43. C. Colón-Emeric et al., "Developing a Process Evaluation Measure of Nursing

Home Care Quality Using Qualitative Case-Study Data," *The Gerontologist* 46, no. Special Issue 1 (2006): 391.

44. K. N. Corazzini et al., ""The Golden Rule": Only a Starting Point for Quality Care," *Director* 14, no. 1 (2006): 255, 257-259-293.

45. R. A. Anderson et al., "Theoretical Overview of Mindfulness and Qualitative Description of Mindful Management Practices in Nursing Homes," *The Gerontologist* 47, no. Special Issue 1 (2007): 54.

46. C. Colón-Emeric et al., "The Impact of Regulation on Mindful and Routine Behavior in Nursing Homes," *The Gerontologist* 47, no. Special Issue 1 (2007): 54.

47. K. Corazzini et al., "The Impact of Professional Nursing Jurisdiction Over Care on Mindfulness in Nursing Homes," *The Gerontologist* 47, no. Special Issue 1 (2007): 54.

48. M. L. Piven et al., "Paying Attention: A Leap Toward Quality Care," *Director* 15, no. 1 (2007): 58-63.

49. R. A. Anderson et al., "Improving Nursing Home Care: Connecting Care & Outcomes Through Local Interactions," *The Gerontologist* 44 (2005): 323.

50. K. Weick, K. M. Sutcliffe, and D. Obstfeld, "Organizing and the Process of Sensemaking," *Organization Science* 16, no. 4 (2005): 409-421.

51. R. A. Anderson et al., "Mindful Management Practices in Nursing Homes," *The Gerontologist* 47, no. Special Issue 1 (2007): 53-55.

52. R. A. Anderson, C. A. Allred, and F. A. Sloan, "Effect of Hospital Conversion on Organization Decision Making and Service Coordination," *Healthcare Management Review* 28, no. 2 (2003): 141-154.

53. R. R. McDaniel, "Chaos and Complexity in a Bioterrorism Future," in *Advances in Health Care Management*, ed. J. D. Blair, M. D. Fottler, and A. C. Zapantam., vol. 4 (Oxford: Elsevier, Ltd., 2004).

54. D. P. Ashmos et al., "What a Mess: Participation As a Simple Managerial Rule to Complexify Organizations," *Journal of Nursing Administration* 39 (2002): 189-206.

55. D. P. Ashmos, D. Duchon, and R. R. McDaniel, "Physicians and Decisions: A Simple Rule for Increasing Connections in Hospitals," *Healthcare Management Review* 25, no. 1 (2000): 109-115.

56. D. P. Ashmos, J. W. Huonker, and R. R. McDaniel, "Participation As a Complicating Mechanism: The Effect of Clinical Professional and Middle Manager Participation on Hospital Performance," *Healthcare Management Review* 23, no. 4 (1998): 7-20.

57. A. F. Tallia et al., "7 Characteristics of Successful Work Relations," *Family Practice Management* 13, no. 1 (2006): 47-50.

58. C. K. Stroebel et al., "How Complexity Science Can Inform a Reflective Process for Improvement in Primary Care Practices," *Joint Commission Journal of Quality and Patient Safety* 31, no. 8 (2005): 438-446.

59. D. Cohen et al., "A Practice Change Model for Quality Improvement in Primary Care Practice," *Journal of Healthcare Management* 49, no. 3 (2004): 155-168.

60. L. M. Leykum et al., "Organizational Interventions Employing Principles of Complexity Science Have Improved Outcomes for Patients With Type II Diabetes," *Implementation Science* 2, no. 1 (2007): 1-8.

61. L. M. Issel and R. A. Anderson, "Intensity of Case Managers; Participation in Organizational Decision Making," *Research in Nursing & Health* 24, no. 5 (2001): 361-372.

A Physicist Looks at Physiology
by Bruce J. West

If we are to understand how the wirewalker retains his
or her balance on the wire, we must analyze the fluctuations, that is, the wirewalker's fine tuning to losses of
balance.[1]

Introduction

Science is not the only lens available for viewing the world around us,
but it has proven, over the past few hundred years, to be among the
most consistent. By this I mean that two individuals viewing the same phenomenon may, within certain limits, obtain similar results. I almost said
they would draw similar conclusions, but this need not be the case. Per-
forming an observation is analogous to doing an experiment, whereas
drawing a conclusion from an observation is applying a theory to the experimental results. These are the two prongs with which scientists attempt
to skewer nature: theory and experiment. But theory and experiment are
only useful when they are under control, meaning that all steps in an experiment are well established and reproducible, and likewise, all elements
of a theory are explicit and internally consistent.

The paradigm of science, since the time of Sir Isaac Newton, has been physics, which entered this world as natural philosophy. As a branch of philosophy, physics was only one of many roads to understanding the physical world. However, with its nearly compulsive reliance on measurement and quantification, its unfaltering determination to give these measurements mathematical expression, and its unwavering attempts to predict the future, physics shed its philosophical association and became the only source of knowledge in the modern world. Or at least that is the view of many. However, physics over the last few decades has run into some difficulties regarding its status as the one true way of knowing the nature of the world. Some of these difficulties are technical, having to do with the mathematics used to model physical phenomena. Other troubles are more systemic and have to do with the interpretation of data, but the two are not unrelated.

The body's healthy operation was in certain respects thought to be similar to a thermodynamic steady state in which health is intolerant of perturbations.

What is most remarkable is that when the foundations of physics began to show cracks, the other sciences, to which the previously believed bedrock ideas of physics had been applied, began to crumble altogether. Physics sneezed and the other sciences got pneumonia. One such application is the concept of homeostasis in medicine. The human body is physical and as such, it is subject to all the laws of the physical sciences. Consequently, for the past two hundred years, medical phenomena have been considered understood to the extent that the underlying physical/chemical mechanisms determining their operation could be made explicit. The guiding principle for this determination was homeostasis—the idea that any disruption in the smooth operation of the body would of necessity be attenuated by the body's natural proclivity to suppress erratic behavior. The body's healthy operation was in certain respects thought to be similar to a thermodynamic steady state in which health is intolerant of perturbations. Furthermore, when the body's health was jeopardized, which is to say, homeostasis ceased to function effectively, then a healthcare professional should intervene to reestablish regularity. In this perspective, disease is just this—the loss of the regularity that homeostasis seeks to maintain.

So what is wrong with this picture? The nurse measures the heart rate, blood pressure, and weighs the patient. But what information about the overall health of the patient does the nurse intend to extract by means of these measurements? For example, one would think heart rate and blood pressure provide indicators of the health of the cardiovascular system at this point in time. But do they? Why do we rely on time-averaged quantities to characterize systems as complex as the cardiovascular, the respiratory, and others? I contend that the distortion of the information wanted and needed for the diagnosis of a patient was and is due to a misapplication of the historical phenomenology of physics.

Consider, for example, the mechanical ventilation of a patient after a surgical procedure. The purpose of ventilation is, of course, to assist the patient in maintaining regular breathing while recuperating from the operation. The regularity of the mechanical ventilator is consistent with the mechanical paradigm that developed from the laws of physics. The problem with this application of the physics paradigm is that healthy people do not breathe regularly. Instead, each breath differs from the last, sometimes being a little faster and sometimes being a little slower. This natural variability, until recently, was considered by the medical community to be part of the noisy background of biological systems and therefore it could and should be ignored. Recent research, however, shows that this biological variability is as important, if not more important, than the average breathing rate. For a more in-depth discussion, see, *Fractal Physiology and Chaos in Medicine*[2] or *Where Medicine Went Wrong*.[3] In the context of ventilation, Alan Mutch, who replaced the historically periodic motion of the mechanical ventilator with the natural variability of a healthy person's respiratory network, established the importance of variability clinically.[4] The improved outcome obtained by using biologically variable ventilators over the controlled ventilators is discussed after we examine the reasons why this should be true.

A Change in Perspective

In the seventeenth century it was impossible to exactly reproduce experimental results. No matter how careful the experimentalist, or how refined the experimental apparatus, the outcome of ostensibly identically prepared, successive experiments gave different results. Usually, the scatter among the outcomes was not very great, but it was always there and could not be avoided. Many methods were developed to explain these fluctuations. The most prevalent was to throw away data too different from the majority as being produced by uncontrolled and therefore unimportant mechanisms. It was the nineteenth century before the German mathematician J. Gauss (1777-1855) identified the arithmetic average as the *best* representation of the results of an ensemble of experiments. Gauss proved that the fluctuations in experimental results were random, but not arbitrary, so that the ensemble could be characterized by a distribution with a bell shape, often called the *normal curve*, with its peak located at the average value. Each experimental result was then either a little larger or a little smaller than the average value, with most results being in the vicinity of the curve's peak. The curve represented the relative frequency of results of a given size occurring in a large number of experiments.

A more subtle application of Gauss' ideas is the measures of health in medicine. The heart rate, breathing rate, blood pressure, and other such averages have long been considered to be the best representations of the corresponding fluctuating physiological systems.

Most results were in the vicinity of the average value and the width of the bell curve determined how unlikely a deviation of a given size was in the ensemble of measurements. Large deviations from the average occurred with less and less frequency as the deviation size increased, as is shown in Figure 1.

The ideas of Gauss found fertile ground in the machines and medicine of the nineteenth and twentieth centuries. From the tolerance of a crankshaft to the quality control of an assembly line, the artifacts of the machine age lent themselves to the description of Gauss. A more subtle application of Gauss' ideas is the measures of health in medicine. The heart rate, breathing rate, blood pressure, and other such averages have long been considered to be the best representations of the corresponding fluctuating physiological systems. The use of these averages in medicine overlooked variability. This view is consistent with the notion of homeostasis, which is seen as the body's natural ability to suppress variability to recapture optimal performance.

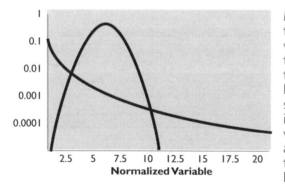

Figure 1: Two kinds of distribution functions are graphed versus a normalized variable, that is, the variable divided by the standard deviation, on log-linear graph paper. The bell-shaped distribution of Gauss is seen to peak at the average value and fall precipitously away from this value, whereas the inverse power law of Pareto goes on and on.

After 200 years of investigation, we are clear about the properties of systems described by the distribution of Gauss. First of all, such networks are linear, so a system's response is proportional to the perturbation. A ten percent excitation produces a ten percent response, or maybe a twenty percent response, but nothing too crazy. The network does not become unstable and therefore, in principle, its behavior can be predicted, at least in a fairly narrow, probabilistic sense. I will probably be as healthy tomorrow as I am today. Second of all, such networks are additive, they can be reduced to fundamental elements which weakly interact and recombine to constitute the overall network. The principle of reductionism operates in full force at the smallest level so fluctuations at the largest scales are produced by variations at the smallest scales, which percolate up into the bell-shaped distribution. Consequently, linear additive phenomena that are stable when exposed to perturbations describe the world of Gauss and homeostasis is a natural consequence of this world-view.

However, what I argue is that this is not the world in which we live. Our world is much more complex than that envisioned by Gauss and there is more than ample evidence to prove it. At the end of the nineteenth century, Vilfredo Pareto, an engineer by training and vocation, took a position as an economist at the University of Laussane, Switzerland, and began his study of society, which for him consisted of politics and economics. Pareto believed that in order to understand the political and economic nature of society, one ought to rely on data rather than philosophical speculation, the latter being the more accepted approach of the time. He applied principles from the physical sciences to the social sciences and in so doing made a discovery that today's scientists are still trying to understand. Scientists are still trying to reconcile the findings of Pareto with the way they would like the world to be.

Pareto gathered data on the distribution of income from a number of western countries and made the remarkable discovery that like the fluctuations in experimental results, the incomes in various countries all satisfy the same law. The law was not the bell-shaped curve of Gauss, however, but something more exotic. The number of people having a certain income level in a given country was found to be proportional to a mathematical power of the level of income. This distribution of income is contrasted with the distribution of Gauss in Figure 1. It is evident from the figure that long after the bell curve predicts that the phenomena should have zero variability, the inverse power law of Pareto predicts substantial activity. In contrast, the distribution of height within a society is a well-known bell-shaped distribution, so the likelihood of someone having a height more than twice the mean is very small. On the other hand, the likelihood of someone having an income twice the mean is substantial, or even ten, a hundred, or thousand times the mean. Consequently, the distribution of income is fundamentally different from that of height. The differences between the distributions of Gauss and Pareto are very dramatic and lead one to very different world-views and specifically different views of physiology and healthcare.

Our world is much more complex than that envisioned by Gauss and there is more than ample evidence to prove it.

If income data are plotted on doubly logarithmic graph paper, the result is a straight line with a negative slope, an example of which is give in Figure 2 for the United States, circa 1918. The straight-line curve (line segments) through the data points has become known as Pareto's Law and, as I said, this law specifies an inverse power-law distribution. An inverse power law income means that the percent change in the population having a certain level of income is proportional to the percent change in the level of income. The proportionality constant between the two quantities is the slope of the inverse power-law curve.

A surprisingly large number of phenomena in the social sciences give rise to Pareto's distribution. Plotting the relative number of times a given word appears in a book written in English versus the rank-order of that word in the book (most frequent, second most frequent, and so on) yields

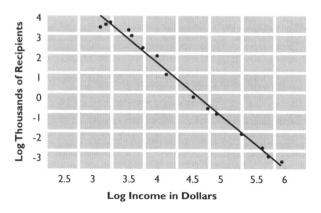

Figure 2: The inverse power law distribution is obtained by plotting the relative frequency of the occurrence of a given outcome, in this case the number of people with a given income level compared with the total population, versus the magnitude of that outcome, here the level of income, on log-log graph paper.[2] The straight line-segment is the best fit to the data points.

an inverse power-law distribution known as Zipf's Law. Graphing the number of cities within a country having a certain population versus the rank-order of that city yields Auerbach's Law. Recording the number of scientists having a given number of publications versus the number of publications produces an inverse power law called Lotka's Law. The Citation Law is an inverse power law obtained from graphing the number of published scientific papers that have a given number of citations versus the number of citations, and of course, Pareto's Law on the distribution of income. These examples have been drawn from sociology, but there are an equal number from botany and biology, for example: the genre containing a given number of species versus the number of species produces Willis' Law; the number of bronchial airways of a given diameter plotted versus the generation number* in the lung was found to be inverse power law by West et al.[5] What distinguishes these processes from one another is the slope of the curve (line-segment) in Figure 2. Only limitations of space restrict the listing of hundreds of phenomena that give rise to inverse power-law distributions.

One mechanism for producing an inverse power law can be identified by comparing two processes operating within the same organism or or-

---

* Each successive branching of a bronchial airway is called a generation, with the trachea being generation zero.

ganization. Suppose each of the two processes has a different growth rate that changes over time, but the changes are such that the ratio of growth rates remains constant. The result will be an inverse power law relating the two processes with a slope determined by the ratio of the two growth rates. This comparison produced the allometric growth laws in biology, as defined by Equation 1[6] and is easily generalized to the social context. The term allometric means by a different measure, so an allometric growth law compares the relative growth rates of two parts of an organism (organization). Suppose we record the number of patients in an Emergency Care Unit (ECU) who occupy a bed for a given length of time. The percent change in the number of people staying in the ECU for a certain time interval is found to be proportional to the percent change in the length of time spent in bed, see, for example, ref.[7]

Complexity is, in fact, the usual situation in physiology/pathophysiology and in healthcare, so we ought not to expect that the associated time series separate into signal and noise.

Here again, the proportionality constant between the two percentages is the slope of the curve relating the two quantities and yields the index in an inverse power-law distribution for the length of stay in the ECU.

Physiology and Homeostasis

The linear additive worldview of Gauss leads to an interpretation of biological time series* that fits the engineering paradigm of signal plus noise. The signal plus noise paradigm is depicted in Figure 3. The signal is assumed to be the smooth, continuous, predictable, and large-scale motion in a time series. A time series can be an electrocardiogram (ECG), an electroencephalogram (EEG), or any other recorded physiologic measurement that changes over time. The idea of a signal and predictability go together, so we anticipate that the heart rate of a healthy individual remains constant unless the body undergoes a stress of some kind. Noise, on the other hand,

---

* A time series is a sequence of measured values of an observable from the system of interest. One can think of the measured values as a dependent dynamic variable, such as CO_2 concentration in the blood, and time as the independent variable. Such series can be either continuous or discrete.

is a typically discontinuous, small-scale, erratic motion that disrupts the signal. The noise is assumed, by its nature, to contain no information about the network, but rather to be a manifestation of the influence of the unknown and uncontrollable environment on the network's dynamics. Noise is considered to be undesirable and is filtered out of the time series whenever possible. The engineering model does not take into account the possibility that the underlying process can be complex and such complexity does not allow for this neat separation into the traditional signal and noise. Complexity is, in fact, the usual situation in physiology/pathophysiology and in healthcare, so we ought not to expect that the associated time series separate into signal and noise. The signal plus noise paradigm does not apply to either physiological or organizational signals in general because of the complexity of the underlying phenomena, complexity that is often manifest in the fractal properties of the time series, as described below.

The fractal concept was formally introduced into science by Benoit Mandelbrot more than twenty years ago, and has since captured the imagination of a generation of scientists. His monograph[8] brought together mathematical, experimental, and physical arguments that undermined the traditional picture of the physical world and supported the empirical studies of Pareto. The work of the mathematician Poincaré on nonlinear dynamical systems in the latter part of the nineteenth century[9] came to be called chaos in the latter part of the twentieth century.

At the time of Poincaré's analysis, the perspective regarding physiology in the medical community was that of homeostasis, which asserts that

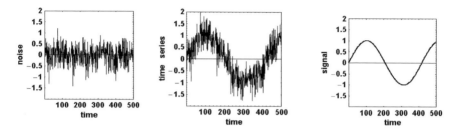

Figure 3: A schematic depiction of a time series in the signal plus noise paradigm. The noise is the fast erratic time series, the signal is the slow smoothly varying time series and the superposition of the two supposedly gives a "realistic" time series.

physiological systems operate in such a way as to maintain a constant output, given a variable input. This vision of the how the body operates dates from the middle nineteenth century and views the human body as consisting of feedback loops and control mechanisms that guide the perturbed physiology back to an equilibrium-like state of dynamic harmony. So the concept of homeostasis must be altered to accommodate the transition of the world perspective from that of Gauss to that of Pareto. In Cannon's book, *The Wisdom of the Body*,[10] he emphasized that the way in which the human body reacts to disturbance and danger maintains the stability necessary for life. Cannon's emphasis was on stability and much of his book recorded the clinical justification for a particular kind of stability. Recent research indicates that this picture is less viable today and a more complete description of physiologic systems requires the use of nonlinear, dynamical concepts and non-stationary statistics, both of which may be manifest through the scaling behavior* of physiological time series

Living organisms are immeasurably more complicated than inanimate objects, which partly explain why we do not have available fundamental laws and principles governing physiological phenomena equivalent to those in physics.

Mandelbrot[3,11] catalogued and described dozens of physical, social, and biological phenomena that cannot be properly described using the familiar tenants of dynamics from physics. The mathematical functions required to explain these complex phenomena have properties that for a hundred years had been categorized as mathematically pathological. Mandelbrot argued that, rather than being pathological, these functions capture essential properties of reality and are therefore better descriptors of the real world than are the traditional analytical functions of nineteenth-century physics and engineering.

Living organisms are immeasurably more complicated than inanimate objects, which partly explain why we do not have available fundamental laws and principles governing physiological phenomena equivalent to

---

*The notion of scaling, described more fully subsequently, implies that what occurs on one scale entails what occurs on another scale. The coupling in allometric growth laws is one example of scaling.

those in physics. Any strategy for understanding physiology must be based on a probabilistic description of complex phenomena and, as we shall see, on our understanding of phenomena lacking characteristic time scales, that is, on self-similar or fractal scaling.

There are three types of fractals that appear in the life sciences: geometrical fractals, that determine the spatial properties of the tree-like structures of the mammalian lung, arterial and venous systems, and other ramified structures;[2] statistical fractals, that determine the properties of the distribution of intervals in the beating of the mammalian heart, breathing, and walking;[12] finally, there are dynamical fractals that determine the dynamical properties of systems having a large number of characteristic time scales with no one scale dominating.[13] In the complex systems found in physiology, the distinctions be-

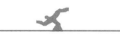

The human body may be seen as a system of systems, each separate system being complex in its own right, but contributing to a complex network of interacting networks.

tween these three kinds of fractals blur, but we focus our attention on the dynamical rather than the geometrical fractals, in part because the latter have been reviewed in a number of places and we have little to add to that understanding.[14]

The description of a complex system consists of a set of dynamical elements, whatever their origin, together with a defining set of relations among those elements. The dynamics and the relations are typically nonlinear. A physiologic system may be identified as such because it performs a specific function, such as breathing or walking, but each of these functional systems is part of a hierarchy that together constitutes the living human body. Consequently, the human body may be seen as a system of systems, each separate system being complex in its own right, but contributing to a complex network of interacting networks. The cardiovascular system, the respiratory system, the central nervous system, and the immune system are all examples of this principle.

Scale invariance is the property that relates the elements of time series across multiple time scales and has been found to hold empirically for a number of complex phenomena, including many of physiologic origin. Consider the scale for a time series, which is determined by the resolving power of a piece of equipment. A scale invariant time series would be one that had the same form independently of whether the unit of measurement was a millisecond, a second, a minute, or an hour. This is also called scaling. The term scaling denotes a power-law relation between two variables x and y, as demonstrated in Equation 1:

Equation 1:

$$y = Ax^\alpha$$

Barenblatt explained this[15] in his excellent inaugural lecture before the University of Cambridge in 1993. He pointed out that such scaling laws are not merely special cases of more general relations. They never appear by accident and they always reveal self-similarity—a very important property of the phenomena being studied. In biology, the relationship described by the above equation (1) is historically referred to as an allometric relation between two observables. Such relations were introduced into biology in the nineteenth century to interrelate the growth of animals and the individual organs.

Physiological Time Series

Herein the allometric relation denoted by Equation 1 is extended to include measures of time series. In this extended view y is interpreted to be the variance and x the average value of the quantity being measured. The fact that these two central moments (measures) of a time series satisfy an allometric relation implies that the underlying time series is a fractal random process. In this section we show that fractal random processes describe all physiologic time series for which there are data.*

Heart Rate Variability (HRV)

For centuries it has been taught that the time interval between beats of the human heart is constant, producing *normal sinus rhythm*. However, measurements by many investigators over the past two decades have shown

---

* Parts of this section are taken from ref. 2.

that this is not the case. In fact, there is a great deal of change in the time interval from beat to beat, even when an individual is resting quietly. The mechanisms producing the observed variability in the size of a heart's interbeat intervals apparently arise from a number of sources. The sinus node (the heart's natural pacemaker) receives signals from the autonomic (involuntary) portion of the nervous system which has two major branches: the parasympathetic, whose stimulation decreases the firing rate of the sinus node, and the sympathetic, whose stimulation increases the firing rate of the sinus node pacemaker cells. The influence of these two branches produces a continual tug-of-war on the sinus node, one decreasing and the other increasing the heart rate. It has been suggested that it is this tug-of-war that produces the fluctuations in the heart rate of healthy subjects. Consequently, HRV provides a window through which we can observe

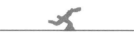

For centuries it has been taught that the time interval between beats of the human heart is constant, producing normal sinus rhythm. However, measurements ... have shown that this is not the case.

the heart's ability to respond to normal disturbances that can affect its rhythm. The clinician focuses on retaining the balance in regulatory impulses from the vagus nerve and sympathetic nervous system, and in this effort requires a robust measure of that balance.[16] A quantitative measure of HRV time series, such as the fractal dimension, serves this purpose.

Consider the beat-to-beat intervals shown in Figure 4a, a typical HRV time series for a healthy young adult male. The data points in the figure are connected to aid in visualizing how the time intervals between heartbeats are changing. It is evident that the variation in the time intervals between heartbeats is relatively small, the mean being 0.72 seconds and the standard deviation being 0.1 seconds. This relatively modest variance seems to support the frequently used medical term *normal sinus rhythm*. So what we learn by plotting the standard deviation and average as a function of resolution of the time intervals is important.

In Figure 4b, the logarithm of the standard deviation is plotted versus the logarithm of the average value for the HRV time series depicted in Figure 4a. At the left-most position, the data point indicates the standard deviation and average using all the data points. Moving from left to right, the next data point is constructed from the time series with two nearest-neighbor data points added together resulting in half the number of data points from which the mean and variance are calculated. The procedure is repeated moving right until the right-most data point has twenty nearest-neighbor data points added together. The solid line segment is the best linear representation of the scaling and intercepts most of the data points with a positive slope of 0.76. We can see that the slope of the HRV data is midway between the dashed curves depicting an uncorrelated random process (*slope* = 1/2), and one that is deterministically regular (*slope* = 1).

We emphasize that the conclusions drawn here are not from this single figure or set of data presented. These are representative of a much larger body of work. The conclusions are based on a large number of similar observations[17] made using a variety of data processing techniques, all of which yield results consistent with the scaling of the HRV time series indicated in Figure 4b. The heartbeat intervals do not form an uncorrelated random sequence. Instead, the analysis suggests that the HRV time series is a statistical fractal, indicating that heartbeats have a long-time memory.

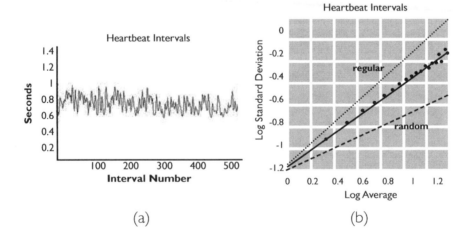

(a)   (b)

Figure 4: (a) The time series of heartbeat intervals of a healthy young adult male is shown. (b) The logarithm of the standard deviation is plotted versus the logarithm of the average value for the heartbeat interval time series for a young adult male, using sequential values of the aggregation number. The solid line segment is the best fit to the aggregated data points and yields a fractal dimension of D = 1.24 midway between the curve for a regular process and that for an uncorrelated random process as indicated by the dashed curves.

The implications of this long-time memory concerning the underlying physiological control network are taken up subsequently.

Phenomena obeying scaling relations, such as shown for the HRV time series data in Figure 4b, are said to be self-similar. The fact that the standard deviation and average values change as a function of aggregation number implies that the magnitudes of these quantities depend on the size of the ruler used to measure the time interval. Recall that this is one of the defining characteristics of a fractal curve—the length of a fractal curve becomes infinite as the size of the ruler used to measure it goes to zero. The dependence of the average and standard deviation on the ruler size, for a given time series, implies that the statistical process is fractal and consequently, defines a fractal dimension for

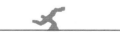

The fractal character of HRV time series emphasizes the non-homeostatic physiologic variability of heartbeats.

the HRV time series. These results are consistent with those first obtained by Peng et al.[18] for a group of ten healthy subjects having a mean age of forty-four years, using ten thousand data points for each subject. They concluded that the scaling behavior observed in HRV time series is adaptive for two reasons: first, that the long-time correlations constitute an organizing principle for highly complex, nonlinear processes that generate fluctuations over a wide range of time scales; and second, the lack of a characteristic scale helps prevent excessive locking into one mode of operation that would restrict the functional responsiveness of the organism.

The fractal character of HRV time series emphasizes the non-homeostatic physiologic variability of heartbeats. Longer time series than the one presented here clearly show patchiness associated with the fluctuations, a patchiness that is usually ignored in favor of average values in traditional data analysis. This clustering of the fluctuations in time can be syptomatic of the scaling with aggregation observed in Figure 4.

Figure 5 depicts HRV time series data for three patients. The top curve is for a normal, healthy individual whose time series has a fractal dimension in the interval $1.1 \leq D \leq 1.3$, empirically determined to be the range of HRV in healthy individuals. The two arrows indicate two different ways the heart can fail to perform its function. The arrow going to the left draws attention to a HRV time series that is nearly periodic, and like the quote

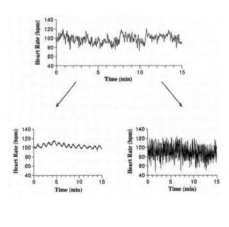

Figure 5: A typical HRV time series with a fractal dimension in the interval $1.1 \leq D \leq 1.3$ is depicted by the upper curve. This is considered normal variability. Two pathology branches emanate from this time series. The one on the lower left has a fractal dimension approximately 1.0 and displays a loss of randomness as seen in conditions such as congestive heart failure, aging, ventricular tachycardia. The time series in the lower right displays a loss of regularity as seen in atrial fibrillation. The fractal dimension is approximately 1.5 (taken from Goldberger[1] with permission)

from the third century Chin Dynasty: "If the pattern of the heartbeat becomes regular as the tapping of a woodpecker or the dripping of rain from the roof, the patient will be dead in four days."[19]

This time series is from a patient with congestive heart failure, and the corresponding fractal dimension is nearly one, which is the fractal dimension of a regular curve. This is the kind of mode locking that was referred to above. The arrow pointing rightward indicates a much different kind of behavior. Rather than becoming more regular, the time series becomes more random. This HRV time series is from a person experiencing atrial fibrillation, and the fractal dimension is nearly 1.5, the same as that for an uncorrelated random process.

These extremes in Figure 5 emphasize two of the dominant pathologies associated with the breakdown of the cardiovascular system. One is the complete loss of randomness, leading to death due to regularity. The other is the complete loss of regularity, leading to death due to randomness. A healthy cardiovascular system cannot survive without a balance of control between the regular and the random. Either one alone is apparently fatal.

Breathing Rate Variability (BRV)

The second physiologic exemplar is the dynamics of breathing—the apparently regular breathing as one sits quietly reading this chapter. To understand the dynamics, we first acknowledge that evolution's design of the lung may be closely tied to the way in which the lung carries out its function. It is not by accident that the cascading branches of the bronchial tree become smaller and smaller, nor is it good fortune alone that ties the dynamics of our every breath to this biological structure. We argue that, like the heart, the lung is made up of fractal processes, some dynamic and others now static. However, both kinds of processes lack a characteristic scale and a simple argument establishes that such a lack of scale

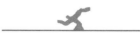

A healthy cardiovascular system cannot survive without a balance of control between the regular and the random. Either one alone is apparently fatal.

has evolutionary advantages and leads to fractal evolution in biology.[20]

Breathing is, in part, a function of the lungs, whereby the body takes in oxygen and expels carbon dioxide. The smooth muscles in the bronchial tree are innervated by sympathetic and parasympathetic fibers, much like the heart, and produce contractions in response to stimuli such as increased carbon dioxide, decreased oxygen, and deflation of the lungs. Fresh air is transported through some twenty generations of bifurcating airways of the lung, during inspiration, down to the alveoli in the last four generations of the bronchial tree. This is an example of a geometric fractal. At this tiny scale there is a rich capillary network that interfaces with the bronchial tree for the purpose of exchanging gases with the blood.

Szeto et al.[21] made an early application of fractal analysis to fetal lamb breathing. The changing patterns of breathing in seventeen fetal lambs and the clusters of faster breathing rates, interspersed with period of relative quiescence, suggested to them that the breathing process was self-similar. The physiological property of self-similarity implies that the structure of the mathematical function describing the time series of interbreath intervals is repeated on progressively shorter time scales. Clusters of faster rates were seen within the fetal breathing data, what Dawes et al.[22] called breathing episodes. When the time series were examined on even finer time scales, clusters could be found within these clusters, and the signature of this scaling behavior emerged as an inverse power-law distribution of time intervals. Consequently, the fractal scaling was found to reside in the statistical properties of the fluctuations and not in the geometrical properties of the dynamic variable. This is an example of a statistical fractal.

As with the heart, the variability of breathing rate using breath-to-breath time intervals is denoted by BRV to maintain a consistent notation. Examples of HRV and BRV time series data on which scaling calculations are based are shown in Figure 6a. Because heart rate is higher than respiration rate in the same measurement epoch there is a factor of five more data for HRV than there are for BRV time series. We have adjusted the scales

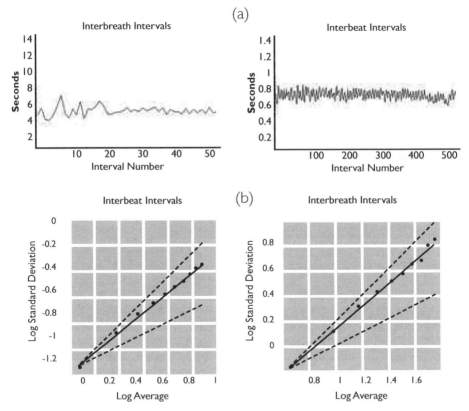

Figure 6: (a) Typical time series from the study conducted by West et al.[19] is shown for the interbreath intervals (BRV) and the interbeat intervals (HRV) time series. Not all the data are shown, just enough to indicate the relative quality of the two time series. (b) The points are calculated from the data and the solid line segment is the best least-square fit to the HRV data (*slope = 0.80*) and to the BRV data (*slope = 0.86*).

in the two graphs to highlight their differences. Looking at these two time series together, one is struck by how different they are. It is not apparent that both physiologic phenomena scale in essentially the same way, but they do.[20]

West et al.[23] analyzed the various HRV and BRV time series and obtained the typical results depicted in Figure 6. Note that we stop increasing the resolution at ten points because of the small number of data in the breathing sequence. The solid line segment at the right in Figure 6b is the best least-square fit to the aggregated BRV data and has a slope of 0.86, the scaling index. A similar graph is constructed for the HRV data in the left curve, where we obtain a slope of 0.80 for the scaling index. The latter slope is so different from that obtained in Figure 4b because of the age difference in the two subjects. The scaling indices and fractal dimension obtained from these curves are consistent with the results obtained by other researchers.

Such observations regarding the self-similar nature of breathing time series have been used in medical settings to produce a revolutionary way of utilizing mechanical ventilators, as mentioned earlier. Historically, ventilators have been used to facilitate breathing after an operation and have a built-in frequency of ventilation. Mutch et al.[24] have recently challenged the single-frequency ventilator design by using an inverse power-law spectrum of respiratory rate to drive a variable-rate ventilator. They demonstrated that this way of supporting breathing produces an increase in arterial oxygenation over that produced by conventional control-mode ventilators. This comparison indicates that the fractal variability in breathing is not the result of happenstance, but is an important property of respiration. A reduction in variability of breathing reduces the overall efficiency of the respiratory system.

Both blood flow and ventilation are delivered in a fractal manner, in both space and time, in a healthy body. However, as Mutch points out,[4] during critical illness, conventional life support devices deliver respiratory gases by mechanical ventilation, or blood by cardiopulmonary bypass pump in a monotonously periodic fashion. This periodic driving overrides the natural fractal operation of the body and Mutch speculates that these devices result in the loss of normal fractal transmission and consequently the damage such life support systems produce increases with increasing use. He goes on to hypothesize that the loss of fractal transmission moves the network through a critical point; one which transforms a cohesive whole into a collection of organ systems that are not well connected.[24]

Altmeier et al.[25] measured the fractal characteristics of ventilation and determined that not only are local ventilation and perfusion highly correlated, but they scale as well. Finally, Peng et al.[26] analyzed the BRV time series for forty healthy adults and found that under supine, resting, and spontaneous breathing conditions, the time series scale. This result implies that human BRV time series, like HRV time series, have long-time correlations across multiple time scales, and therefore breathing is a fractal statistical process.

Stride Rate Variability (SRV)

Walking is one of those things we do without giving it much thought, day in and day out. We walk confidently with a smooth pattern of strides and without apparent variation in gait. The regular gait cycle, so apparent in everyday experience, is not as regular as we believed. Gait is no more regular than is the normal sinus rhythm or breathing just discussed. The random variability observed in stride intervals is so small, however, that the biomechanical community has historically considered these fluctuations to be an uncorrelated random process. In practice this means that the fluctuations in gait were thought to contain no information about the underlying motor control process. Consequently, in the design of rehabilitation protocol, only the average gait is considered and not the natural variability of walking. In this way, treadmills became the technique of choice, just as did the control-mode mechanical ventilators discussed above. A revolution in rehabilitation awaits the champion who introduces normal biological variability into the protocol, in the same spirit as Mutch has done in ventilation.

One hundred years after the first experiments to quantify the degree of irregularity in walking, the follow-ups were finally done. In the middle of the last decade, Hausdorff et al.[27] observed the stride intervals of healthy individuals, as well as those of subjects having certain neurophysiologic disorders, such as Parkinson's and Huntington's disease, that affect gait and the elderly. West and Griffin[28] did additional experiments and analyses, which both verified and extended the earlier results.

Like normal sinus rhythm in the beating of the heart, where the interval between successive beats changes, the time interval for a gait cycle fluctuates in an erratic way from step to step. The gait studies carried out to date concur that the fluctuations in the stride-interval time series exhibit long-time inverse power-law correlations indicating that the phenomenon of walking is a self-similar fractal activity.

One definition of the gait cycle or stride interval is the time between successive heel strikes of the same foot.[24] An equivalent definition of the stride interval uses successive maximum extensions of the knee of either leg.[4] The stride interval time series for a typical subject is shown in Figure 7 where it is seen that the variation in time interval is on the order of three to four percent, indicating that the stride pattern is very stable. Here again, for name consistency, we indicate time series for the stride intervals by stride rate variability (SRV). It is the stability of SRV that historically led investigators to decide that not much could go wrong by assuming the stride interval is constant and the fluctuations are merely physiological noise. The experimental data fluctuations around the mean gait interval, although

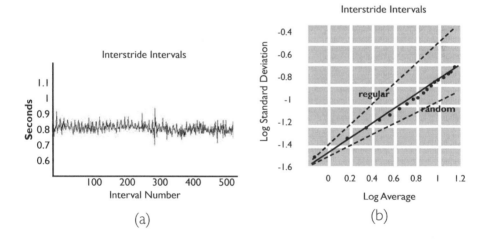

(a)   (b)

Figure 7: (a) The time interval between strides for the first 500 steps made by a typical walker in an experiment[24] is depicted. (b) The logarithm of the aggregated standard deviation is plotted versus the logarithm of the aggregated mean, starting with all the data points at the lower left to the aggregation of 20 data points at the upper right. The SRV data curve lies between the extremes of uncorrelated random noise (lower dashed curve), and regular deterministic process (upper dashed curve) with a fractal dimension of $D = 1.30$.

small, are non-negligible because they indicate an underlying complex structure and as we show, these fluctuations cannot be treated an uncorrelated random noise.

Using as SRV time series of fifteen minutes, from which the data depicted in Figure 7a were taken, we analyze the data to determine the scaling index from the time series as shown in Figure 7b. The slope of the data curve is 0.70, midway between the two extremes of regularity and uncorrelated randomness. So, as in the cases of HRV and BRV time series, we again find the erratic physiological time series to represent a random fractal process. In the SRV context, the implied clustering indicated by a slope greater than the random dashed line, means that the intervals between strides change in clusters and not in a uniform manner over time. This result suggests that the walker does not smoothly adjust his or her stride from step to step. Rather, there are a number of steps over which adjustments are made followed by a number of steps over which the changes in stride are completely random. The number of steps in the adjustment process and the number of steps between adjustment periods are not independent. The results of a substantial number of stride interval experiments support the generality of this interpretation.

Once the perspective that disease is the loss of complexity has been adopted, the strategies presently used in combating disease must be critically examined.

The elderly are often prone to falling down without any apparent reason. Whether this loss of grace is a consequence of inattentiveness, or whether it is due to something more basic, such as a neurodegeneration, remains unclear. What is clear is that the scaling of the SRV time series for seniors, when compared with young adults, changes dramatically. Hausdorff et al.[27] determined that, on average, seniors and young adults have virtually indistinguishable average stride intervals and required almost identical lengths of time to perform standardized functional tests of gait and balance. This lack of difference is not unlike the average heart rates, where the average heart rate ceases to be a useful indicator of cardiac pathology. However, the scaling indices of these two groups indicated that the stride interval fluctuations are more random and less correlated for the elderly than for the young. This loss of long-time memory in the elderly arises even though the magnitude of the stride-to-stride variability is very similar for the two groups. Consequently, the gross measures of gait and mobility function do not seem to be affected by age, whereas the scaling exponent clearly changes with age.

Subjects with Huntington's disease, a neurodegenerative disease of the central nervous system, also presented a reduction in the scaling exponent below that of a disease-free control group. The control group had an index in the same range as the youths above, whereas the group with Huntington's disease had a scaling parameter equivalent to the aged. The control and Huntington's groups were chosen to be equivalent to one another, in that they were not statistically different in terms of gender, height or weight. Another curious result was that the severity of the disease increased inversely with the scaling parameter, that is, the memory of the fluctuations of the SRV time series decreases with increasing severity of the disease, where the severity is scored using an established measure known as the total functional capacity score of Unified Huntington's Disease Rating Scale. Consequently, the increasing severity of Huntington's disease is measured by the decreasing complexity of the body's gait system.

Conclusions

We have seen that although physiologic time series, such as the interbeat intervals of the human heart, the interstride intervals of human gait, and the interbreath intervals in human breathing, are apparently random, they do, in fact, have long-time memories. This combination of randomness and order has been used herein as the defining characteristic of complexity. In a medical context this complexity is encountered when attempting to understand physiological phenomena from a holistic perspective, rather than looking at specific mechanisms. Analysis establishes that such dynamic physiologic phenomena generate time series that are statistical fractals. The scaling behavior of such time series determines the overall properties such complex networks must have and they are not like the older analyses of errors and noise in physical systems.

The historical view of complexity involved having a large number of variables, each variable making its individual contribution to the operation of the network and each variable responding in proportion to the changes in the other system variables. Small differences in the input could be washed out in the fluctuations of the observed output. The linear additive statistics of measurement error or physiological noise is not applicable to the complex medical phenomena discussed here. The elements in complex physiologic systems are tightly coupled, so instead of a linear additive process, nonlinear multiplicative statistics more accurately represent the fluctuation, where what happens at the smallest scale can and often is coupled to what happens at the largest scale. This coupling is manifest here through the scaling index.

Once the perspective that disease is the loss of complexity has been adopted, the strategies presently used in combating disease must be critically examined. Life support is one such strategy, but the tradition of life support is to supply blood at the average rate of the beating heart, to ventilate the lungs at their average rate and so forth. Blood flow, ventilation, and other physiologic processes normally operate in a fractal manner, in both space and time, in a healthy body. As discussed, the periodic driving of the life support networks overide the natural aperiodic operation of the body. A similar observation may be made regarding physical therapy where the periodic nature of the treadmill is supposed to strengthen the muscles used in such normal activities as walking.

A number of scientists have demonstrated that the stability of hierarchical biological networks is a consequence of the interactions among the elements of the network. Furthermore, there is an increase in stability resulting from the nesting of networks within networks—organelles into cells, cells into tissues, tissues into organs, and so on up from the microscopic to the macroscopic. Each network level confers additional stability on the overall fractal structure. The fractal nature of the network suggests a basic variability in the way networks are coupled together. For example, the interaction between cardiac and respiratory cycles is not constant, but adapts to the physiologic challenges being experienced by the body.

To paraphrase West and Griffin,[24] the signal plus noise paradigm used by engineers is replaced in physiology with the paradigm of the high-wire walker. In the circus, high above the crowd and without a net, the tightrope walker carries out smooth average motions plus rapid erratic changes of position, just as in the signal plus noise paradigm. However, the rapid changes in position are part of walker's dynamical balance, so that far from being noise, these apparently erratic changes in position serve the same purpose as the slow graceful movements, to maintain the walker's balance. Thus, both aspects of the time series for the wirewalker's position constitute the signal and contain information about the dynamics. Consequently, if we are to understand how the wirewalker retains balance on the wire, we must analyze the fluctuations, that is, the wirewalker's fine tuning to losses of balance as well as the slow movements. This picture of the wirewalker more accurately captures the view of biological signals developed herein.

Bruce J. West, PhD, FAPS, FARL, is chief scientist at the Mathematical & Information Science Directorate of the Army Research Office. His research focus has been on the development of the mathematical tools necessary to understand complex phenomena. His work on the fractional calculus for the modeling of complex phenomena lead to Physics of Fractal Operators (with Bologna and Grigolini, Springer, 2003) for which he received the Army Research Laboratory Award for Publication in 2003. As exemplars of complex networks, he has pursued research in physiology and the modeling of nonlinear biomedical phenomena leading to the books *Biodynamics: Why the Wirewalker Doesn't Fall* and *Where Medicine Went Wrong*. Dr. West has authored more than 350 publications.

Works Cited

1. B. J. West and L. A. Griffin, *Biodynamics Why the Wirewalker Doesn't Fall* (Hoboken: Wiley-Liss, 2004), 4.

2. B. J. West, "Fractal Physiology and Chaos in Medicine," *Studies of Nonlinear Phenomena in Life Science* 1 (1990).

3. B. J. West, *Where Medicine Went Wrong: Rediscovering the Path to Complexity* (Singapore: World Scientific, 2006).

4. A. Mutch, "Health, 'Small-Worlds', Fractals and Complex Networks: An Emerging Field," *Medical Science Monitor* 9, no. 5 (2003): MT55-MT59.

5. B. J. West, V. Bargava, and A. L. Goldberger, "Beyond the Principle of Similtude: Renormalization in the Bronchial Tree," *Journal of Applied Physiology* 60 (1986): 1089-1098.

6. J. S. Huxley, *Problems of Relative Growth* (New York: Dial Press, 1931).

7. P. Philippe, M. R. Garcia, and B. J. West, "Evidence of 'Essential Uncertainty' in Emergency Ward Length of Stay (EWLS)," *Fractals* (2004): 197-209.

8. B. B. Mandelbrot, *Fractals, Form, Chance and Dimension* (San Francisco: W.H Freeman and Co., 1977).

9. H. Poincaré, "Mémoire Sur Les Courves Définies Par Les Equations Différentielles," *Gauthier-Villars* I-IV, no. 1 (1888).

10. W. B. Cannon, *The Wisdom of the Body* (W.W. Norton, 1932).

11. B. B. Mandelbrot, *The Fractal Geometry of Nature* (San Francisco: W.H. Freeman and Co., 1982).

12. B. J. West and W. Deering, "The Lure of Modern Science: Factal Thinking," *Studies of Nonlinear Phenomena in Life Science* 3 (1995).

13. B. J. West, "Physiology, Promiscuity and Prophecy at the Millenium: A Tale of Tails," *Studies of Nonlinear Phenomena in Life Science* 7 (1999).

14. P. Meakin, "Fractals, Scaling and Growth Far From Equilibrium," *Cambridge Nonlinear Science Series* 5 (1998).

15. G. I. Barenblatt, *Scaling Phenomena in Fluid Mechanics* (Cambridge: Cambridge University Press, 1994).

16. M. Marek et al., "Heart Rate Variability: Standards of Measurement, Physiological Interpretation, and Clinical Use," *European Heart Journal* 17 (1996): 354-381.

17. B. Suki et al., "Fluctuations, Noise and Scaling in the Cardio-Pulmonary System," *Fluctuations and Noise Letters* 3 (2003): R1-R25.

18. C. K. Peng et al., "Long-Range Anticorrelations and Non-Gaussian Behavior of the Heartbeat," *Physical Review Letters* 70 (1993): 1343-1346.

19. Y. C. Liu, *The Essential Book of Traditional Chinese Medicine* (New York: Columbia University Press, 1988), 4.

20. B. J. West, "Physiology in Fractal Dimension: Error Tolerance," *Annals of Biomedical Engineering* 18 (1990): 135-149.

21. H. H. Szeto et al., "Fractal Properties of Fetal Breathing Dynamics," *Regulatory, Integrative and Comparative Physiology* 32 (1992): R141-R147.

22. G. S. Dawes et al., "Respiratory Movements and Rapid Eye Movement Sleep in Fetal Lambs," *The Journal of Physiology* 220 (1972): 119-143.

23. B. J. West et al., "The Independently Fractal Nature of Respiration and Heart Rate During Exercise Under Normobaric and Hyperbaric Conditions," *Respiratory Physiolgy & Neurobiology* 145 (2005): 219-233.

24. W. A. C. Mutch et al., "Biologically Variable Ventilation Increases Arterial Oxygenation Over That Seen With Positive End-Expiration Pressure Alone in a Porcine Model of Acute Respiratory Distress Syndrome," *Critical Care Medicine* 28 (2000): 2457-2464.

25. W. A. Altemeier, S. McKinney, and R. W. Glenny, "Fractal Nature of Regional Ventilation Distribution," *Journal of Applied Physiology* 88, no. 1551 (2000): 1557.

26. C. K. Peng et al., "Quantifying Fractal Dynamics of Human Respiration: Age and Gender Effects," *Annals of Biomedical Engineering* 30 (2002): 683-692.

27. J. M. Hausdorff et al., "Altered Fractal Dynamics of Gait: Reduced Stride-Interval Correlations With Aging and Huntington's Disease," *Journal of Applied Physiology* 82 (1997): 262-269.

28. B. J. West and L. Griffin, "Allometric Control, Inverse Power Laws and Human Gait," *Chaos, Solitons & Fractals* 10, no. 1519 (1999): 1527.

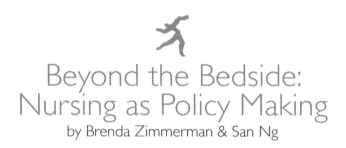

Beyond the Bedside:
Nursing as Policy Making
by Brenda Zimmerman & San Ng

Act like a nurse but think like a movement.
– *Brenda Zimmerman*

Palliative Care: A Nurse-Led Global Movement

The modern North American palliative care movement is often credited to the work of Dr. Cicely Saunders, a nurse, social worker, and physician, and Florence Wald, Dean of Nursing in the 1960s at Yale. In 1963, Yale's medical school invited Saunders from London to give a presentation to the medical faculty and students. Wald heard of Saunders' visit and asked if Saunders would repeat the presentation to the nursing students and faculty. Wald listened attentively as Saunders described her work in Britain. "To us she was a nurse, and [palliative care] was the epitome of nursing," Wald said. "It was a very, very moving experience for me."[1] It changed her life. Within a few years of hearing Saunders' speech, Wald had resigned as Dean to found the first hospice program in North America. Later she turned her attention to prison hospice services.

Wald had become increasingly frustrated with the dominance of the curative role of medicine in the 1960s. Historian Arnold Toynbee said

"Death is un-American – an affront to the American dream." The 1960s was a time of the civil rights movement and the sexual revolution. The palliative care movement, although quieter and more subtle, was also raging against the norms of the day. This movement was challenging the foundations of modern American medicine. Death, like sex, was a taboo topic for discussion prior to the 1960s. Civil rights and patient rights shared some fundamental challenges in overthrowing dominant approaches in society. "In 1963 we were struggling with patients, particularly the cancer patients, who were being treated with surgery and with radiation in the hospital," Wald recalled. "And despite the fact their condition was worsening, curative treatment was pursued."[1]

Although palliative care had its roots in the nineteenth century, it was the work of Saunders and Wald that brought it to the forefront. Saunders began changing policy for patients in her own hospital in the late 1940s. Later, her efforts spread to the regional, national, and international stages, in large part through the work of Florence Wald. The changes in care and the health policies generated had a rather inauspicious beginning in an encounter with a patient. David Tasma, a Polish Jew dying of rectal cancer in a busy London teaching hospital, touched Saunders emotionally. He knew he was dying and wanted to ensure that his illness and death would benefit others.

Saunders was deeply moved by the fact that David knew he was dying, yet the hospital was only organized for cure, not for care. Her deep sadness about David's treatment began a lifelong quest to discover ways that dying people could be treated with dignity and relief from pain. Saunders developed new methods of medical pain management, promoted psychological wellbeing through hospice-style care and appropriate counseling, and created both social and spiritual support networks to provide end of life care. Saunders also understood that this care needed to be supported by research that demonstrated the benefits of palliative care, and increased the legitimacy and visibility of the movement. To this end, in 1967, she opened Saint Christopher's Hospice in south London as the first academic hospice where patients could go for relief of "total pain," including its physical, psychological, social, and spiritual dimensions. In addition, nurses and doctors working in the hospice could study this work in a rigorous fashion and add to both the applied and published knowledge of palliative care.[2]

Health policy can be defined as a course of action that influences healthcare decisions. By this definition, Cicely Saunders and Florence Wald were major policy figures of the twentieth century. Their work, both at the bedside and in the hospices, region, country, and eventually the globe, has shaped and continues to shape resource allocation decisions, physician and nurse education, research agendas, and more. "What I have found is that people can die in good health," Wald said.[1]

Are Cicely Saunders and Florence Wald anomalies or is there something intrinsic to nursing that is linked to policy? In this chapter, we argue that although Saunders and Wald are exceptional, nurses' participation in policymaking is not. The nursing profession has always played a key role in health policy. The challenge is both to remind nurses of how powerful their influence can be in policy and to reflect on how nurses should think about policy creation. This is where a complexity-inspired approach provides new insights.

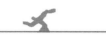

The nursing profession has always played a key role in health policy. The challenge is both to remind nurses of how powerful their influence can be in policy and to reflect on how nurses should think about policy creation.

The Calling of Nursing

Many nurses come to their profession through a calling—to improve care for patients and populations. The calling is often extremely local—to help individual patients and their loved ones deal with the challenges of illness. But nurses are also drawn to their profession because of their desire to prevent illness and to create more caring contexts for all citizens. Nurses, often intuitively and through training, come to understand how local and more *global* needs are connected. The calling is one that addresses populations even while serving individuals.

Once inspired nursing students become nurses, they face the political and cultural realities of healthcare in an era of cost containment, cutbacks, and nursing shortages. Many begin to feel constrained, powerless, and frustrated. These frustrations often lead nurses to avoid broad issues and focus instead on immediate tasks and individual patients. In essence, the calling that originally drew them to nursing can become muted under the pressures of the daily work and the politics of healthcare. This chapter provides a ray of optimism for nurses and proposes that a focus on national and international issues using complexity-inspired approaches can remind nurses of their calling and enable them to have a more significant impact.

This chapter addresses three questions:

- Why should nurses and nurse educators care about policy, especially policy related to national and international issues?

- How is a complexity-inspired approach to healthcare policy different from the dominant healthcare policy rhetoric and practice?

- How can Complexity Science help nurses impact the important health policy issues?

As is obvious by the nature of our questions, the bias brought to this chapter is that nurses can and do influence health policy, and that insights from Complexity Science provide an opportunity to address some of the most challenging health policy issues faced by nurses and the larger healthcare community.

Complexity Science and the Misleading Language of "Systems"

Every nurse is familiar with the term *system* and more particularly *healthcare system*. It is common parlance to use phrases such as "the system is broken," "national health systems," and "integrated healthcare systems." And yet the term system has radically different meanings in the dominant and Complexity Science-informed perspectives. Understanding health policy, a course of action that influences healthcare decisions, from radically different "systems" perspectives can guide nurses' actions and reflections on their actions. Table 1 outlines the different concepts of policy when we view healthcare as a "mechanistic system" versus a "complex system."

For many, the term "system" has been wedded to an implicit mechanistic metaphor. Replace the word system with machine and the meaning of the common phrases in the paragraph above changes little for many. But by using the word system, the underlying metaphor and its implica-

Table 1: Healthcare policy – two conceptions of systems

Systems as Machines view	Complex Systems view
Perspective of Policy	
• External perspective "The system, the environment" • Primary focus on the individual parts versus the connections between the parts • Patterns primarily examined within levels • Needs to be highly structured	• Embedded perspective "Within our system, of our system" • Focus on relationships among the parts • Patterns repeat across levels • May be loosely structured
Policy Planning	
• Large-scale plans • Blueprint for what needs to be done • Predictable, rational, linear forecasting • Legislation to define details of behavior– regulations and prescriptions	• Small-scale plans, seeding across the system • Emergence, learn as you go • Unpredictable and nonlinear and therefore may use scenario planning or multiple experiments • Legislation which outlines principles or boundaries
Policy Implementation	
• Top-down direction • Carry out prescribed plans (planners separate from implementers) • Large-scale changes • Imposed consistency (external), limit variability • Best practice (for replication) • Linear, carry out plan • Both ways (top-down and bottom-up)	• Planning and actions are iterative (planning and implementation are embedded) • Small-scale changes • Inherent coherence (patterns that repeat and enhance) so allow for diversity, positive deviance • Nonlinear, don't have to just carry out plan, also try new things
Policy Evaluation	
• Compliance, gold standard, generalizable • Quantifiable, measurable outputs	• Effectiveness for local context (context specificity) • Qualitative, focus on learning and development as an output—use of evaluation to understand how outcomes (qualitative and quantitative) were achieved

tions are buried. The view of "system as machine" suggests that one can fix it—the parts (often called "human resources") need to be understood and fixed or replaced. One can reengineer the system and its parts, and one can be separate from the machine while fixing it. Knowledge becomes a manageable, separate entity[3]* and its "mechanics" can be studied in order to make improvements. This dominant view of systems has influenced policy makers both in terms of how they create policy and the content of the policies created. It has also influenced how nurses conceive of their role in national and international policy issues.

Believing implicitly in a system as machine, nurses would see the policy making framework as separate from their daily work, and that it should involve rational planning, forecasting, and predictions. Nurses would look for the blueprint, ask "who is driving the bus?" and expect large-scale plans to trigger large-scale changes. Good policy would be generalizable and result in imposed consistency across the board. Nurses would ask for or participate in the creation of coordinating mechanisms, nurse-to-patient ratios, and human factors engineering to address patient safety and quality. From this machine perspective, there is said to be a need to create *standardized* systems of care and *consistency* across nations about immunization practices, HIV/AIDS treatment, and other important health issues.[5] Legis-

---

* Ralph Stacey and his colleagues Patricia Shaw and Douglas Griffin have taken this idea of systems one step further. They argue by viewing organizations as systems we are trapped into a view of the world which limits our understanding of how knowledge is created. The systems view sees knowledge more as a thing that is situated in an individual's brain. Instead they offer an alternative to systems thinking by arguing that knowledge is not a thing that can be situated but rather "an ephemeral, active process of relating" (Stacey, 2001, p4). Instead of talking about complexity as complex adaptive systems, they refer to complex responsive processes. We are very sympathetic to their perspective. However, in trying to bring Complexity Science ideas into the policy realm, we believe the first step is to move people away from a mechanistic view of systems to a biological perspective. Once we have made that move, the more radical move to complex responsive processes can naturally follow. But we are concerned that given the conservative nature of policy making in North America, we still need to use some language that they can connect with and "systems" is the ubiquitous term. In some ways our approach is less authentic than that of Stacey and his colleagues because we are embedding complex responsive processes ideas into the traditional "systems" language. Yet, we believe this subversive approach is needed at this stage of policy development to be heard and hence have an impact.[3,4]

lation is often sought which defines specific courses of action in terms of regulations and prescriptions. The challenge for nurses interested in policy is not to throw out these ideas. For some issues and some contexts, mechanistic approaches are powerful. It is important to recognize, however, that the metaphor underlying these interventions and policies is limiting when dealing with the human endeavor of health and healthcare.

For complexity scientists, the concept of a system is drawn from biological metaphors and suggests evolving and growing rather than "fixing." Humans are not resources but interacting, continuous co-creators of knowledge and understanding. Relationships are the key focus rather than the individual "parts." Emergence and unpredictability are inherent and ubiquitous, and one can never be outside of a system because of the embedded nature of complex adaptive systems (CASs). This biological view of complexity and systems is in stark contrast to the machine metaphor.

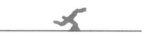

Believing implicitly in a system as machine, nurses would see the policy making framework as separate from their daily work, and that it should involve rational planning, forecasting, and predictions.

Believing in the biologically inspired systems view, which is central to Complexity Science, requires a radical rethinking of how policies are created (a descriptive stance) and should be created (a normative stance). Policy would not be seen as externally derived, but rather derived from an embedded perspective where all nurses are "of" the system. Emergence and unpredictability would be expected, and considered to add value in many contexts. Planning and implementation would be iterative rather than separate processes. Locally derived, specific solutions would create an inherent coherence across the system rather than an imposed consistency. Dershin advises that it is futile to try to manage complex organizations through such methods as strategic planning and "top-down" rulemaking. He states that such methods do not work in chaotic environments because small differences in the environment can lead to large differences in outcomes. Dershin also states that local circumstances are important and management must recognize and adapt to these circumstances.[6]

Complexity Science asks us to pay attention to how coordination of care naturally occurs and the social processes that create coordination.

Rather than set staffing ratios, which assume a "nurse is a nurse is a nurse," implying interchangeable "parts," we need a deeper understanding at a local level of what makes for effective, efficient, caring, and healing contexts. Legislation is designed to outline principles and boundaries within which innovations can thrive. The boundaries create limits to behavior but also allow for freedom of action within the boundaries. Details of behavior are left to local design. Rather than employing human factors engineering, which looks at humans as having faults such as memory lapses, we look to how human interactions contribute to an increase in safety. In other words, we look to the very nature of human relationships and interactions as the source of quality. Since we can never be outside of the system, we look to include patients, their families, clerical, and cleaning staff into the patient safety and quality discussion.

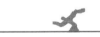

Complexity Science asks us to pay attention to how coordination of care naturally occurs and the social processes that create coordination.

Florence Wald understood these ideas deeply. The team approach, including the patient, family, professionals, and staff providers, was central to her model. Some of the requirements to work in her original hospice in New Haven, Connecticut, included a strong foundation in basic nursing skills, flexibility, and the ability to provide emotional support and education to patients and families. Today, nursing is still the primary source of professional services in palliative care. "Hospice nurses work interdependently with other members of the team."[7] However, they also function independently when the local context—the needs of the patient and families—calls for interventions to address pain, social, psychological, and spiritual issues.[7] The dance steps between interdependence and acting locally are deeply wedded to an understanding of human relationships and interactions.

Wald began her journey into palliative care because of a particular concern for cancer patients. She saw how curative approaches came at the expense of care and nurturing. Cure was winning in the tug-of-war between cure and care. Her work brings the two closer together in terms of their impact on patients. Today, her original concern for understanding patients with cancer and their families continues to ripple through the nursing profession.

Complexity Science is about relationships—including the deeply human relationships that impact outcomes and quality. It calls us to be more attentive to naturally occurring solutions and to use these in our repertoire to improve patient care.

Positive Deviance (PD) is one way to discover and amplify local solutions. PD is a development approach that is based on the premise that solutions to problems already exist within communities that have problems. Hence, it challenges the traditional, externally driven approach to development and problem solving. It is closely linked with Appreciative Inquiry.[8-10] The idea of deviance is that the behavior is outside of the norms of the community

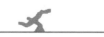

Complexity Science is about relationships — including the deeply human relationships that impact outcomes and quality.

or group studied. PD is the term used to describe abnormal practices or behaviors that lead to positive outcomes. The approach has been used extensively in developing countries to understand how some infants become better nourished and healthier than the average despite experiencing the same poverty as their neighbors, and in amplifying the practices that produce the better outcomes. PD seeks to work with the existing resources rather than looking to external sources. The main features of the PD approach fit well with Complexity Science perspectives that systems are embedded in local context, outcomes are emergent and unpredictable, knowledge is specific versus generalizable, and connections or relationships shape behavior.

Current Model of Policy for Nursing

A conceptual model of nursing and health policy developed by Russell and Fawcett,[11] and subsequently expanded[12] provides a comprehensive depiction of the current perspectives of policy for nursing. This conceptual model has been well received in nursing and was ranked as the ninth most frequently cited article in *Policy, Politics and Nursing Practice* as of July 2, 2005.

Three sources of nursing health policy are considered by the model: 1) *public policies* are those that are developed by nations, states, cities, and towns, and typically have a broad impact on individuals, groups, organizations, and communities; 2) *organizational policies* are developed by healthcare facilities, such as hospitals, clinics, and home healthcare agencies, to guide practice at a particular institution; 3) *professional policies* are the standards and guidelines developed by nursing-specific and multidisciplinary associations that provide guidance to the profession. Any of these sources can have an impact on healthcare services, healthcare personnel, and healthcare expenditure policies.

Russell and Fawcett's[12] model comprises four interacting levels, each addressing one or more of the main elements of health policy: quality, cost, and access to health services:

- *Level 1*. Emphasizes the health policy concept of quality by addressing the efficacy of nursing practice processes on the health and wellness of individuals, families, groups, and communities

- *Level 2*. Emphasizes the health policy concepts of quality and cost by addressing the effectiveness of nursing practice processes and the effectiveness and efficiency of healthcare delivery subsystems on health outcomes

- *Level 3*. Emphasizes the health policy concept of access by addressing societal demands for quality of access to effective nursing practice processes and efficient nursing practice delivery systems, as well as equity in the distribution of the costs and burdens of care delivery

- *Level 4*. Emphasizes the health policy concepts of quality, cost, and access by addressing the issue of justice and the social changes that are required to facilitate allocation of high-quality, cost-effective, healthcare services and other health-related resources

This model clearly defines the elements that need to be considered in developing and applying health policy, a hallmark of the approach to policy driven by the machine metaphor (for instance, identifying the parts). However, the model also goes beyond identifying the elements of the system to suggest that there are different levels of health policy that may interact with each other. In addition, the model suggests that one level of policy focus is not better than another, but rather as one progresses from the first to the fourth level, the policies become increasingly broad. That is, the model does not characterize health policy impacts as being top-down or bottom-up, but rather bidirectional. This conceptualization of nursing policy is consistent with a key principle of Complexity Science (embeddedness). It has been used for nursing education in the United States[13] and has been applied to analyze policies regarding various nursing issues.[14-19]

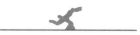

Paying attention to a broader spectrum of Complexity Science principles creates some new foci for health policy.

Although this conceptualization of policy addresses some of the key elements of complexity, including embeddedness and micro-macro connectedness, it does not address others such as emergence, unpredictability, relationships, and nonlinearity. Paying attention to a broader spectrum of Complexity Science principles creates some new foci for health policy. In effect, by more explicitly incorporating a complexity theoretical framework, insights into new interventions become apparent, as previously "hidden" complexity variables are brought to the foreground.

What Does Complexity Science-Informed Policy Look Like?

Return now to the story of the palliative care movement. If we looked at the story from a Complexity Science perspective, what would we notice or pay attention to as we tried to understand the policy impact of the movement?

Saunders had the capacity to see her patient, David Tasma, not only as an individual but as an indicator of what was not working well in healthcare. Saunders and Wald built on these ideas and revealed how the dominant patterns and modes of connecting with patients were neglecting a whole group of patients who would always exist—dying patients. They were able to see how the macro (global trends, especially in modern western medicine) and meso levels (national and regional policies in addition to resource allocation decisions) impacted the local levels (hospital and direct patient care) and vice versa. Their learning from one level influenced the other levels, both up and down.

Wald and Saunders saw the power of embeddedness. They were explicit that a dying patient's care was embedded in the hospital system, family context, and the spiritual beliefs of patients and providers. The palliative care movement uses the term "hospice," derived from the Latin noun meaning both host and guest, implying relationship and mutuality. As a guest, one cannot impose treatments but can be welcomed by a host to participate in care as mutually defined and created. Saunders and Wald were comfortable with the ambiguity of simultaneously being a host to their patients and a guest in their lives. This capacity to embrace ambiguity and paradox is also a cornerstone of complexity.

The palliative care movement is about locally derived solutions. It is a prime example of coherence without the need for consistency. Coherence suggests that you can recognize the care as palliative because of a few key values and attributes. However, palliative care is not a blueprint. There is no consistency among patients. Each palliative care situation is a negotiated relationship between patient, family, volunteers, and clinical caregivers. Research and external evidence is gathered, not to prescribe set standards, but to provide insights into what could be included effectively in the care regime. Creativity and respect for local knowledge are consistent with Complexity Science.

Palliative care is the antithesis of "a nurse is a nurse is a nurse." Instead, it focuses on caring relationships that will make a person's last days comfortable and address their emotional, physical, and spiritual needs. The role of the nurse will depend on a wide variety of factors in the existing relationships the patient has with family, friends, and volunteers.

The content of palliative care policy is consistent with many of the principles of Complexity Science. How about the process? Saunders and her colleagues in the movement learned from the bottom up. They learned from patients and trusted the local knowledge of patients and their immediate care givers. They looked at both clinical literature and experience to determine what already worked. This included medications to reduce pain and bring comfort. It also included creating a context at Saint Christopher's Hospice and New Haven Hospice where they could experiment and learn deeply through action. The hospice movement focused on relationships and how to enhance them. It was understood that emergence and unpredictability would be part of the process, and Saunders and Wald made sure that policies recognized this and allowed for local creativity and variation based on patients' needs. The process embraced paradox—they did not attack the cure approach, but rather found a way to enhance it by providing alternative treatments to cure. Care and cure co-exist.

Contemporary Policy Topics for Nursing

In the following section, we apply the principles of Complexity Science to three major nursing issues of our time: 1) the HIV/AIDS epidemic; 2) global nursing shortages; and 3) patient safety. We discuss how each of these issues would be conceptualized from mechanistic systems and Complexity Science perspectives. Table 2 shows how the mechanistic view and the Complexity Science view differ with respect to these issues. For each issue, we see that shifting the focus to complexity requires us to pay attention to aspects of issues which are often underemphasized in traditional policy perspectives.

HIV/AIDS Global Pandemic

The HIV/AIDS pandemic is the worst health disaster in human history in terms of number of deaths. Although AIDS is now considered a chronic disease in much of the developed world, for the vast majority of the world's population, AIDS remains a death sentence. The extreme differences in treatment availability on a global scale and our seeming tolerance of huge disparities in health are a stain on human history. With this backdrop, nurses across North America have been taking up the gauntlet to address HIV/AIDS at home and across the globe.[20] Nurses, individually and through their professional associations, have gone to some of the worst hit areas of the world to serve the local populations, to train and work alongside local healthcare providers, and to influence regional and national policies. The pandemic is not abating, and the need for nurses to play an active role in all aspects of the disease remains pressing.

Looking at HIV/AIDS with a mechanical systems perspective, it is incumbent upon nurses involved in policy to help create national or international infrastructures. There is a need to have consistent applications or

Table 2: Current policy issues from a mechanistic and complexity perspective

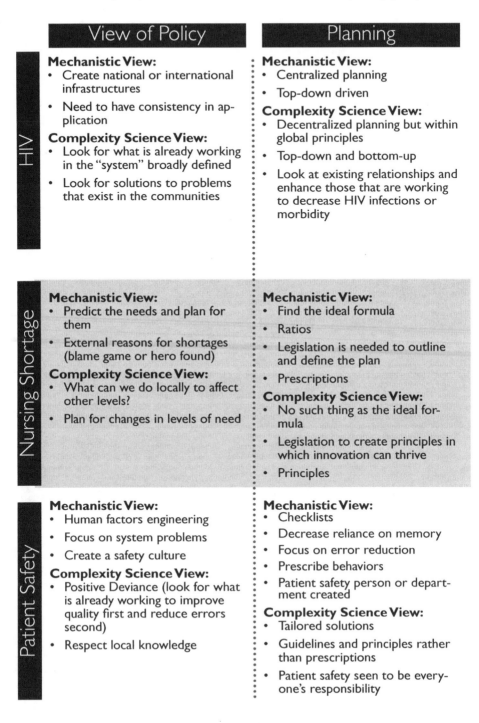

	View of Policy	Planning
HIV	**Mechanistic View:** • Create national or international infrastructures • Need to have consistency in application **Complexity Science View:** • Look for what is already working in the "system" broadly defined • Look for solutions to problems that exist in the communities	**Mechanistic View:** • Centralized planning • Top-down driven **Complexity Science View:** • Decentralized planning but within global principles • Top-down and bottom-up • Look at existing relationships and enhance those that are working to decrease HIV infections or morbidity
Nursing Shortage	**Mechanistic View:** • Predict the needs and plan for them • External reasons for shortages (blame game or hero found) **Complexity Science View:** • What can we do locally to affect other levels? • Plan for changes in levels of need	**Mechanistic View:** • Find the ideal formula • Ratios • Legislation is needed to outline and define the plan • Prescriptions **Complexity Science View:** • No such thing as the ideal formula • Legislation to create principles in which innovation can thrive • Principles
Patient Safety	**Mechanistic View:** • Human factors engineering • Focus on system problems • Create a safety culture **Complexity Science View:** • Positive Deviance (look for what is already working to improve quality first and reduce errors second) • Respect local knowledge	**Mechanistic View:** • Checklists • Decrease reliance on memory • Focus on error reduction • Prescribe behaviors • Patient safety person or department created **Complexity Science View:** • Tailored solutions • Guidelines and principles rather than prescriptions • Patient safety seen to be everyone's responsibility

Implementation	Evaluation
Mechanistic View: • Create new standards of care that are generalizable • Focus on aggressive therapies to attack disease (see disease as separate from social, political, economic web) • Use practices that worked elsewhere **Complexity Science View:** • Experiment and learn with others • Learn from local culture to co-create appropriate care approach • Recognize the interconnectedness of the disease, social, political, and economic contexts • Tailor practices to work locally	**Mechanistic View:** • Randomized control trials as "gold" standard • Generalizable evidence **Complexity Science View:** • Evidence is both locally derived (specific) and general across contexts • Focus on what is being learned and who is learning – need local learning
Mechanistic View: • Apply same formula to each setting – count the nurses as "bodies" • PCS – patient classification systems for ideal staff mix **Complexity Science View:** • Teach staff to regulate work flow based on their knowledge of local context • Use continuous improvement ideas	**Mechanistic View:** • Expect same quality for given formulas • Research findings to create generalizable standards **Complexity Science View:** • Feedback from staff, patients, other stakeholders • Use PCS as benchmark for comparison and to open discussions on how to create optimal mix • Track feedback and patterns of workflow and reactions to it
Mechanistic View: • Documentation • Change the colors of labels, ensure human slips are minimized • Standardization • Routinize • Reduce variability **Complexity Science View:** • Effectiveness focus for local context • Customization • Increase awareness by all staff to focus on quality • Recognize variability as asset	**Mechanistic View:** • Audit • External validation **Complexity Science View:** • Reflection, inquiry, sharing • Self-assessment (skills to do effective self assessment)

policy frameworks around the globe. This requires centralized planning and a top-down approach. Under this perspective, leadership from the top is needed to create meaningful change. New standards of care must be created and implemented across populations. The focus should be on aggressive therapies to attack the disease. Best practices that work in one context would be exported to others. Evaluation would include randomized control studies as the accepted "gold" standard. "Evidence-based" would be interpreted as that which can be generalized.

The mechanistic view of systems is incapable of portraying some of the interdependencies and relationships that are keys to understanding and addressing HIV/AIDS.

Laudable as many of these approaches are, they are not enough. The mechanistic view of systems is incapable of portraying some of the interdependencies and relationships that are keys to understanding and addressing HIV/AIDS. A complexity perspective complements and challenges the mechanistic view. From a complexity viewpoint, the disease cannot be treated in isolation from its social and political context. For example, in the developing world, the disease impacts young women at a much faster rate than men.[21] For this reason, it is critical to understand the gender, culture, and power dimensions that affect incidence, prevalence, and mortality. Treatments and prevention strategies must consider the interconnectedness of these variables. Education, particularly women's literacy, is directly correlated with decreased risk of contracting HIV/AIDS. A Complexity Science perspective would look at the relationships among these variables, and consider what is already working. Working with the positive deviants, the outliers that are creating positive impact can provide leverage to address the challenge and spread locally derived practices that resonate with the cultural, political, and socio-economic conditions.

Policy planning needs to be decentralized to respect local knowledge and traditions. Global and national bodies can be very helpful in providing resources and in creating guidelines or principles that allow for local creativity and adaptability. Nurses, individually and in professional associations, can play a role in demanding that local knowledge be incorporated into policies and that national and international bodies respect local (or specific) knowledge and do not become overly prescriptive in their work. Principles and guidelines are needed. Coherence, which implies an overall pattern that "hangs together," is valued more than consistency. Consistency assumes all should be treated in the same way and thus implies "an AIDS patient is an AIDS patient is an AIDS patient." Such a perspective is not necessarily effective under varying conditions or in different contexts. Coherence implies that equity trumps equality. What is needed are a few key principles that can be applied in many contexts and that allow for translation into locally appropriate actions. Nurses can work with the evaluation aspects of policy to ensure that lessons learned are both local and global. Researchers and care providers from outside the community or country and the researched or the local patients and care providers need to be seen as learning partners. Learning should be co-created within a given context rather than separated from it.

An example of how local knowledge and influence can be tapped to co-create a successful program which addresses HIV/AIDS is shown in the story in Box A.

The Nursing Shortage

Policy related to nursing recruitment and retention is particularly significant in an era of nursing shortages, at local, national, and global levels.[5;22] The existence of a nursing shortage is seen to create a self-perpetuating, vicious cycle. Because there are too few nurses, existing nurses are overworked, frustrated, and may be less motivated to fulfill their calling. This is reported in the press and professional publications, leading to the perception that nursing is a poor job choice for young people. Hence recruitment and retention problems further exacerbate shortages and nurses' frustration. On and on the cycle continues.

Looking at this policy challenge from a mechanistic viewpoint, it is important to predict staffing needs and plan for them. However, in a mechanistic system, there is a sense that one is outside of the system and someone else is in control or "driving the bus." When shortages occur, it is clear that the driver has steered the wrong course. Explanations are based on externalities or the "blame game." The department is short of nurses because the hospital budgeted poorly. The hospital is short of nurses because of poor regional planning. The region is short of nurses because the schools

Box A: Acting locally: HIV/AIDS prevention in South Africa

The following story is told by Brenda Zimmerman and is based on her research on HIV/AIDS in South Africa.

South Africa once had the dubious honor of being the AIDS capital of the world.* In that country, the government went from denying AIDS, to calling antiretroviral drugs "Western poison," to providing these drugs free to its citizens. Understandably, the public, and in particular the women, are suspicious and unclear about what to believe. Western nurses may be viewed with suspicion as they are not deemed to understand local ways of doing things. Knowing that women tend to trust their hairdressers, western and local nurses sponsored by L'Oreal trained South African hairdressers in HIV/AIDS prevention and treatments so the hairdressers could educate their clients. By valuing and understanding local context and identifying the naturally occurring trusted relationships, these nurses created an opportunity to increase the rate of adoption of prevention approaches, testing, and treatment. The hairdressers, unlikely allies in a public health campaign, provided an important service to the community and became a source of information about effective ways to transmit prevention messages. ■

of nursing have not produced enough graduates. The futility of the blame game is evident, often even to those immersed in playing it, yet the mechanistic assumptions lead us to believe there is someone in control.

Mechanistic models would look for an ideal formula to address workforce shortages.[22] Such formulas might include mandatory nurse to patient ratios or patient classification systems (PCSs), that aim to create ideal skill and staffing mixes. Evaluation methods would assume that ratios and PCSs can be applied in a standardized fashion for comparison purposes. One would expect the same quality given the same ratio and PCS.

Complexity scientists looking at nursing shortages would start with a different set of assumptions. First, they would assume that there are likely to be local variations which cannot be captured in the aggregated data of ratios and PCSs. They would also begin with the assumption that the system has embeddedness and that what happens locally can impact what happens at higher levels in the hierarchy as well as vice versa. Rather than looking for the answers from "above," they would look at how local actions affect other levels. For example, recruiting nurses from outside of your normal catchment area could lead to shortages elsewhere. This has been important implications for the practice of recruiting nurses from developing countries. Many professional associations are creating policies aimed at addressing this challenge. Using Complexity Science perspectives, one does not seek a single ideal solution. Instead, one looks for patterns. Positive patterns should be reinforced. Negative patterns should be examined to understand how local actions can effect change.

Rather than imposing formulas such as PCSs and ratios, Complexity Science approaches would suggest that local variation is a source of knowledge and inspiration. Hence, staff should be taught to regulate the workflow based on their knowledge of the local context. Using continuous improvement ideas, nurses should be participating in creating the staffing policies that would best improve patient care.

In poll after poll, nursing ranks at or near the top in terms of most trusted professions, yet burnout and reduced enrollment in nursing programs have affected staffing levels. See the story, *Where's the Care* at the end of this chapter for information on how a nurse administrator at one New Jersey hospital addresses the nursing shortage using Complexity Science Principles.

Patient Safety

Patient safety has become one of the most talked about arenas for health policy in the past decade. Conferences, books, articles, and courses addressing the poor safety record of North American healthcare systems, especially hospitals, proliferate. Steps have been taken to shift attention away from finding the scapegoat or one individual responsible to a systemic view. But the question is which systemic view is being followed, mechanistic or complex? In this chapter we argue that the mechanistic perspective has been predominant. Again, as with the other policy issues, there have been significant gains from applying this orientation but there are also limits. A Complexity Science perspective is an ideal complement to address patient safety in a more comprehensive manner.

The dominant mechanistic approach to patient safety has created the need for a safety culture. To create such a culture, human factors engineering is emphasized.[23;24] Humans are assumed to have slips, trips, and lapses in memory which lead to errors. To overcome the shortcoming of the human machine, there is a need to standardize, routinize, and prescribe protocols and specific behavior, in other words, to engineer. Checklists and physical changes to the layout of rooms, equipment, and medications are designed to address "human machine" errors. Quality is subsumed under the rubric of error reduction and patient safety officers or committees are established and charged with reducing error rates. Variability is seen as an enemy of error reduction and hence it is the job of the patient safety committee to find ways to reduce variability. Audits and external validation of the reduction in errors is a key part of the evaluation.

Surprise, emergence, and variability are not enemies to quality patient care but rather keys to innovation.

These mechanistic approaches have been somewhat effective in reducing some errors. However, these methods may not be sufficiently broad to capture the full spectrum of patient safely issues let alone the broader category of quality. Complexity Science, with its emphasis on the living systems concept, draws attention to aspects of healthcare that are hidden from a mechanistic view. Clinicians are seen not as error producers or faulty machine parts, but as being in relationships with their patients and other care providers. These relationships have the potential to be rich sources of information about what is effective and appropriate in care. Including a broader spectrum of players in efforts to improve quality and safety increases the number of eyes and ears paying attention to emerging patterns. Patients, families, clerical staff, and housekeepers, as well as nurses and other clinicians, are part of the relationship web which co-creates quality and patient safety. The patient safety movement could learn lessons about how to work effectively with these webs of relationships from the work of Florence Wald and her followers in the palliative care movement.

Surprise, emergence, and variability are not enemies to quality patient care but rather keys to innovation. Nurses need to pay attention to surprise, emergence, and variability and incorporate what they learn into their care plans. Paying attention to local solutions and using approaches like PD can provide powerful tools for improving patient care. Hence, policies need to be created that allow for local knowledge to be incorporated into behavior patterns.

Using a PD framework, nurses can look for what is already working to improve quality and reduce errors. Policies that create principles rather than prescriptions and those that incorporate a broad spectrum of stakeholders are also consistent with a Complexity Science orientation. Evaluation should include reflection, story-telling, inquiry into emerging patterns, and sensemaking. Self-assessment approaches need to be developed. For example, consider the following story told to the authors of this chapter by a nurse working on a general surgery ward at a tertiary acute care facility:

> One time I was covering for another nurse while she was on break. She told me that all of her patients were fine and that I could just look into them whenever. Even though I was too busy to keep up with my own patients, I did a walk around. When I glanced into one of her patient's room, my 25 years of nursing experience told me that something was wrong... Sure enough, even though the patient was stable at the time, he took a turn for the worse...he could have died. Others would say 'those aren't my patients, he can wait,' but I don't think that way...

In this case, the patient is seen as central and interactions between nurses and patients, as well as the context of those interactions, are understood as emerging patterns. Humans naturally recognize patterns. In a complex view of patient safety, we want to ensure that we are taking advantage of pattern recognition skills.

Complexity is a powerful perspective for nurses to think about policy. For the issues discussed, existing policy frameworks are dominated by mechanistic models, but often have some complexity aspects as well. However, if the complexity perspective remains hidden, it is our contention that many of its insights will be overshadowed by the more prevalent mechanistic mindset. Nurses can play a key role in shaping policies that embrace complexity principles so that relationships, emergence, and unpredictable aspects of healthcare are examined and developed.

Conclusion

Traditionally, healthcare policy has addressed three realms: healthcare services, personnel, and expenditures. Many times these categories have been seen to be quantifiable or monetizable. In other words, the questions asked within these three categories are often in the form of "How many?" or "What will it cost?" Often, there also is the implicit assumption that policy is created by others and imposed upon a system. Broadly, health policy is about courses of action that influence healthcare decisions. If we are interested in looking at practices that change health outcomes, then we need to be also asking questions that do not lend themselves to prediction and generalizability. Our contention is that much of what we are concerned about in healthcare today is about quality—quality of care for our patients, quality of lifestyle for the healthcare

Although we acknowledge the frustration and feelings of impotence nurses often experience, we believe there is optimism in the Complexity Science perspective.

providers, quality of life for populations, and equity within regions, countries, and the world. Only some aspects of quality are quantifiable and monetizable. Many are more qualitative, relationship based, and context specific. We do not dismiss efforts to quantify but rather want to recognize their limitations for creating and understanding policy. Complexity Science can complement these traditional approaches by drawing attention to relationships, emergence, and local contexts. In doing so it can be used to enhance nursing's influence on health policy. At the end of this chapter is a story written by Roger Lewin and Britue Regine entitled *Where's the Care?* This story describes how nurses from Hunterdon Medical Center in New Jersey and some other facilities utilize Complexity Science principles to address some of the issues discussed in this chapter including relationship-building, the nursing shortage, patient safety, and quality.

This chapter began with the idea that nursing is inherently a call to address policy issues. Although we acknowledge the frustration and feelings of impotence nurses often experience, we believe there is optimism in the Complexity Science perspective. Recognition of nonlinearity (how small differences can potentially have a big impact), embeddedness (how changes at one level can cascade up or down the levels), the importance of specific or local knowledge, and the power of relationships to create conditions for change suggests that nurses in all contexts can contribute to practices that change health outcomes.

Where's the Care?[25]

By Roger Lewin and Britue Regine
(used with permission from Plexus Institute)

It was a simple enough exercise to kick off the meeting proceedings, but one with profound results: "Think back to a time, a single incident, when you felt you were thriving as a nurse," conference participants were instructed. "Now find a partner and tell your story." The energy in the room instantly swelled, as almost a hundred nurse administrator, healthcare researchers and educators relived rich moments that most had not thought about for years. They were moments when these dedicated professionals had felt connected to their calling, connected to what they care about in their work, connected to the care in healthcare. For many, it was a Kleenex moment.

Participants had gathered for three days at Hunterdon Medical Center, in New Jersey, a hospital where care–and even love–is palpable in the corridors. Their mission: to explore "Creating Healthcare Environments Where Nurses Thrive." Nurses obviously thrive at Hunterdon, so there would be lessons to be learned from that. There would also be lessons learned from the sponsor of the gathering, Plexus Institute, a not-for-profit enterprise whose mission is to help communities, organizations and individuals thrive, guided by principles of complexity science. While some people might be set back on their heels by the conflating of "complexity science" and "care," that partnership of words and deeds is, in fact, natural and deep, as participants came to hear and experience.

The context of the gathering was twofold. First, it came in the wake of the Institute of Medicine's 2003 report on patient safety and the work environment for nurses, and a previous Institute study which carried the startling conclusion that upwards of 100,000 patients die in US hospitals each year as a result of medical error. "The healthcare system in this country is broken," said co-convener Linda Rusch in her opening remarks. "Patient safety is a big part of that. This meeting is the beginning of a historical conversation, where we have for the first time nurses, educators, and researchers coming together in the same room since the IOM report, to address patient safety."

The second factor was the current crisis in nursing, a crisis with an odd paradox. On one hand, the nursing profession is judged to be the one most respected of all professions for its ethics and honesty, according to a recent Gallup Poll. Nursing garners an 83 percent approval among the public, compared with 68 percent for medical doctors (number two on the list) and 11 percent for HMO managers. On the other hand, nursing is ranked just 137th out of a list of 250 professions as being a desirable pursuit. Burnout and job dissatisfaction are substantially higher in nursing than most other professions; retention is significantly lower; almost half of new RNs leave within one or two years; enrollment in nursing programs has fallen 22 percent in the past decade; and 54 percent of nurses say they would not recommend the profession to a friend. Clearly, nurses as a whole are not thriving. And, as Marjorie Wiggins, of Maine Medical Center noted, healthcare is headed towards its own version of the perfect storm. "We have hard working professionals trying to deliver a caring service," she told the audience. "They are working in an aged delivery model functioning in a problematic infrastructure. What lies ahead is a known disaster—shortages, decreased reimbursement, increased demand, growing dissatisfaction of care providers—all known to threaten the ability of the system to deliver safe care."

To Rusch, who is VP of Patient Care Services at Hunterdon, the paradox in nurses' work lives offers an opportunity. "I firmly believe that patient safety and nurses' work environment are strongly linked," she said. "When you have a work environment in which nurses thrive, patient safety is improved. When nurses love their jobs, they take good care of their patients. We've all known this intuitively, and now, over the past few years, we've seen research that confirms the link. We know what to do. What is holding us back?" It was a good question, with many answers, one of which is the size and complexity of the healthcare system, where nurses make up almost one quarter of healthcare workers.

The study that got most exposure at the gathering was a survey of the effect of patient load on nurses' burnout and patient safety, led by Linda Aiken, of the University of Pennsylvania, published in the fall of 2002. The conclusion was simple: numbers matter. For instance, when a nurse is responsible for eight patients she (and 95 percent of nurses are women) is more than twice as likely to suffer emotional exhaustion and burnout than a nurse with a four patient load, and almost twice as likely to be dissatisfied with her job. One consequence is that almost half of the nurses who suffer burnout plan to quit within twelve months, as compared with just 11 percent who don't complain of burnout. Sadly, nursing is a caring profession where nurses increasingly lack the time to forge caring relationships with their patients, because of the growing patient load.

Another consequence is more deadly. Exhausted nurses make mistakes, don't catch other people's mistakes, and don't notice when patients are in trouble (failure to rescue). As a result, more patients suffer from preventable conditions, such as deep vein thrombosis, pneumonia, urinary tract infections, and bed sores, all of which extend a patient's length of stay, cause discomfort, and cost the hospital dearly in the purse. Some may even die. According to the Aiken survey, a patient who shares a nurse with seven other patients is 30 percent more likely to die from complications than one who shares a nurse with just three other patients.

In addition to the impact of a heavy patient load, nurses' efficiency and job satisfaction are strongly influenced by the management style they work under. For instance, Ruth Anderson, of Duke University School of Nursing, told the audience of her survey of nursing homes, where management tends to be highly bureaucratic, partly because they are so heavily regulated. "Under this style of management, nurses feel detached from and dissatisfied with their work, and patients suffer frequent falls and often have to be restrained," she said. The survey also included institutions where management was, as Anderson put it, "relationship oriented." By this she meant that managers had good relationships with their staff, were concerned about staff feelings, and included them in decision making. "Under this style of management nurses were more committed to their work, had higher job satisfaction, and there were fewer negative issues with patients."

Similarly, a study of so-called magnet hospitals, where nurses are included in making decisions that affect their work, nurses stay in their jobs an average of eight years, which is twice as long as they do in hospitals where style management is the traditional command and control mode. It's easy to see why nurses typically are excluded from decision making, as revealed by an ANA survey of healthcare professionals: while nurses are regarded as primarily responsible for patient safety, only 8 percent of physicians polled said that nurses should be included in making decisions that govern their work. Physicians' often say that their role is to cure patients, while the nurses are there merely to care for them. That degree of lack of professional respect causes trouble, as a famous study at Beth Israel Hospital, Boston, shows clearly: When nurses don't have good relationships with physicians in the ICU, conflict is high, and mortality rate rises.

Nurses at the conference were brutally honest about another paradox in a profession where care is central to how people are with each other, or should be: nurses too often are mean to each other. Instead of offering support when a colleague is stressed or confused, which happens especially when new RNs face the reality of their profession as compared with what they learned at nursing school, nurses can be unhelpful and rough on each other. "When nurses are upset with a system that is toxic, they turn on each other," says Diana Crowell, a nursing educator at the University of New Hampshire. "It's unfortunate, but it does occur." Linda Rusch describes it as a kick-the-dog syndrome. "You feel abused by the system, so you become an abuser. You don't feel supported, so you don't offer support to colleagues who need it. It's really sad." Sad, yes, and it is little wonder that so many new RNs leave the profession within a year or two, and that retention generally is so low.

What does a complexity science perspective of organizations have to say about these travails? A great deal, because at the heart of the science is the recognition of the positive influence of good relationships among people, and the power of including people on the front line in making decisions that affect them. The science suggests that when a manager attends to the relationships she has with her staff, and when she embraces them in making decisions–part of shared governance–her organization will perform outstandingly, and her people will be committed to their work, and will love their jobs. To many people schooled in the traditional command and control style of management, all this sounds "soft" and "unbusinesslike," and, well, "feminine." But any manager who disdains these simple rules does so at his peril, if efficiency and performance are the goals. There are many organizational development studies that show clearly that relationship-oriented, or feminine, management styles lead to robust bottom line business results.

Hunterdon Medical Center is a beacon in this respect. It is financially healthy, has high patient satisfaction scores, and retention of nurses is well above the national average. Linda Rusch has played no small part in these achievements, as she described in an informal, "living room conversation" format she had with Jim Begun, a healthcare educator at the University of Minnesota, on the conference's opening day. "When I was approached to be VP of Patient Services here a dozen years ago, they said to me, 'We are looking for a healing executive,'" said Rusch. "The previous nurse executive didn't have good relationships with her department heads, and the work environment was quite toxic. Part of my background is in psychology, and that gives me an important skill set, because it is natural for me to want to be in relationships. When I think about what makes me thrive, it is about having good relationships with the people I work with. Of course, there are tough days when I want to pack it in, because of the stress. But, for me, the greatest joy I derive from my job is working with the department heads."

When Rusch arrived at Hunterdon a dozen years ago, she knew nothing about complexity science. Indeed, the science was still in its infancy then, especially in relation to organizational health. Then, ten years ago Curt Lindberg, president of Plexus who was with VHA at the time, gathered healthcare executives together in Philadelphia to ask the question: "Is there a different way of leading?" The intellectual framework of the meeting was complexity science, whose key message to leaders is: "Ease up on the control thing, and you will unleash the creativity in your people." Rusch immediately embraced the new science, because, she says, it is so natural. "It doesn't matter what your scientific background is, many of you know this way of working intuitively. It's nice to have a science that validates this way of working; it's nice to name it scientifically; but it isn't necessary to be able to do it successfully."

Complexity science emerged over the past decade and a half as a way of understanding how the world really works. The prevailing view of nature was very mechanistic, believing that nature is made up of parts, and all you needed to be able to understand how the whole works was to know how the individual parts worked. The essence of this view was that you were in control, everything was predictable, and no surprises. This mechanistic perspective became incorporated into management theory, and is the basis of command and control management. It is true that some of the world is like that, comfortably linear. But most of the world is not like that; it is disturbingly nonlinear, or complex, as anyone who pays attention to the work environment knows all too well. And as Joan Stanley, of American Association of Colleges of Nursing, noted, "Nursing is an extremely complex profession that requires practice within extremely complex organizations and systems."

Instead of viewing organizations as being like machines, which are controllable and predictable, complexity science views them in a much more biological and human framework, as being organic. Organizations, it says, are complex adaptive systems, systems that are finely tuned to external and internal influences, and as a result are constantly adapting. And much of what emerges in this process will be a surprise. Complex adaptive systems are, to use that old adage, more than the sum of their parts, hence the occasional unpredictability of what emerges from them.

Complexity scientists learned from computer models that complex adaptive systems are most adaptable and creative when four things are in place: first, when there is rich interaction between the agents in the system; second, when the agents are free to self organize, rather than be directed all the time; third, when there is constant feedback about what is happening; and fourth, a recognition that small changes can have a big impact on the system, as those changes ripple through the system and build a critical mass for major change. This last of the four is the most counterintuitive, because in the mechanistic model of organizations, major change can be achieved only through major intervention.

Henri Lipmanowicz, chair of Plexus, translated this complexity language into what it means day-to-day for managers and their staff in an organization. Rich interactions among agents equates to good relationships among people. Being free to self-organize means that people on the front lines should have the power to have influence over their work environments, and do what they think is necessary, rather than expecting to be told what to do. It is known as distributed control, as opposed to centralized control. Having feedback requires managers to be constantly vigilant, and to listen to what their staff has to say. Knowing that small changes can have big effects liberates people who are frozen into inaction by the enormity of change that is required in the healthcare system, and encourages them to take small actions among the people around them. "Storytelling is one of the most powerful things you can do in the workplace," Lipmanowicz told the audience. "Remember the first morning when you told your stories. When you do this at work you get strong emotional connections within minutes, and you get a very different kind of information than happens in typical workplace exchanges. That can be a potent engine of change."

Linda Rusch, in her conversation with Jim Begun addressed these practical issues, too. "You establish relationships by really listening to people," she said. "It's not just a perfunctory, 'How are you doing.' It's, 'How was your weekend?.....Tell me about that.'" While many managers are obsessed with controlling their staff, Rusch relishes "unleashing them," as she puts it. "They are out there doing their stuff," she laughs, "and half the time I have no idea what they are doing, until they tell me. They are very, very creative when they work like this." Rusch encourages feedback in several ways. First, there is a monthly meeting called Lessons Learned, at which any issue, thorny or positive, can be brought up with complete honesty, something most managers would shy away from. "You can never learn unless you are willing to be vulnerable," she said. Staff nurses are also present on the hospital's governing council. "That can be uncomfortable for some people," she told the audience. "Not here. We need the staff nurses. We need their knowledge and their experiences, to help shape us." As for making small changes, she encouraged staff nurses to get educated about shared governance, be involved in performance improvement, be a voice for safety, tell stories.

Rusch likens her style of management to being a cultivator and cites a saying from the management theorist Gareth Morgan. "Farmers don't grow crops," she said. "They create conditions for crops to grow. It's the same with people in organizations, and you can have great success. Of course there will always be difficult people, and you have to deal with that. Here at Hunterdon we have a meeting called Liberation, where we talk about difficult people, and find ways of nurturing them, caring for them. But if they don't change their ways, they are assisted in leaving the hospital. You have to take care of the whole organization. It's like pruning diseased branches from a tree, for the sake of the health of the whole plant."

The gathering was about as far from typical conferences as could be imagined. Instead of didactic PowerPoint presentations, much of the activity was around individual participation, beginning with the storytelling exercise. "The purpose," said Lipmanowicz, "was so that you can experience complexity science in action, making the connections, self-organizing, allowing for surprises." But it was just the beginning of a conversation that the conveners plan to nurture in the future. One practical outcome, said Linda Rusch, was a plan to establish learning networks among the participants, and to set up a database where people can post small changes that have been successful, so that others can learn. Another, according to Curt Lindberg, was to work in partnership with the American Association of Colleges of Nursing to integrate complexity science into the clinical nurse leader curriculum. A third outcome, initiated by Michael Bleich, of the University of Kansas School of Nursing, is to devote a single issue of a nursing journal to complexity science, its philosophy and practical application. "By putting all this knowledge and experience in one place, it will be accessible to nursing professionals, whereas now the literature is scattered," said Bleich. "That way we will be able to build a critical mass around this way of working, and help change the healthcare system."

Participants had come to Hunterdon to find ways of creating environments in which nurses can thrive. In a way, they already knew the answer, in the stories they told that first morning, about a time when they personally felt they thrived. Here are a few:

Diana Crowell, healthcare educator, University of New Hampshire: "I went right back to when I was at the bedside, over 20 years ago, and I saw myself in the white uniform and the white shoes, remembering how I would polish them and how good I felt about my work. One night, on a heavy surgical floor, I was going around getting patients settled for the night. This one gentleman was close to being panic stricken about the surgery he was to have the next day. I could see that that wouldn't make him a good candidate for surgery, being in that state. "I told the nurse supervisor that I was concerned, and that I thought he needed more attention. She said to me, 'Go be with him. We'll cover for you, because you are good at helping people with their anxieties.' I sat with him and let him vent his anxiety. I answered practical questions about what was going to happen the next day. I was just with him as a caring human being, letting him feel the care, until after about half an hour or so he drifted off to sleep, no longer anxious."

Ardath Youngblood, perinatal nurse educator, Hunterdon Medical Center: "Hunterdon is a great place to work, but we do have problems, too. Three years ago we had a glitch in the admissions computer system in obstetrics. If a mother comes in and has her baby, everything is fine. But if there is pre-term labor, and the mother is discharged when the baby isn't born, then the next time she's admitted it's as if there is a second baby, according to the computer files. It was very confusing, like having several babies floating around, not linked to the mother. "This one time we admitted a mother who had had pre-term labor a few weeks before. The baby was born this time, a little girl, premature, just three pounds, with respiratory distress syndrome. We took blood for lab work, but then couldn't use it because the computer records were wrong, because of this glitch we have. We called up admissions, very frustrated. They were frustrated as well, a lot of negative conversations going on. Meanwhile, the baby wasn't getting the treatment it needed.

"Stephanie Dougherty from Risk Management said, 'How can this be going on?' Linda Rusch got involved, and finally she said, 'We need to have a meeting to get this thing solved.' Everybody was there, the director of admissions, director of the lab, director of the information systems, etc. It was pretty tense in the beginning. People were saying, 'We can't change the system. It's too complicated.' Everybody was being very defensive. Finally I spoke up, but before I said anything I put the baby's footprints on the table, so that everyone could see them. 'This is what we are dealing with,' I said. 'This tiny baby, every breath she takes her chest collapses. She's crying, grunting. It's awful. And we are supposed to take more blood from her, because of this computer glitch, and she's not getting treated!' "Everybody just became quiet, stopped being territorial and defensive. Instead, they said, 'How can we fix this?' In no time we had the computer record glitch was fixed, and there hasn't been a problem since. For me, the moment was my being listened to in a forum like that, and getting something done that everyone said couldn't be done."

Loraine Skeahan, RN at Hackettstown Community Hospital, NJ: "I had a woman patient with colon cancer, and she was due to go into surgery. Her husband came to me and asked, 'Would it be alright if I played our wedding song, because we'd like to dance one last time before she goes to the OR?' I said, 'OK.' I'm looking at my watch. There wasn't much time. I said, 'First I'll have to make a phone call.' I spoke to the head nurse in the OR, to the surgeon and to the anesthesiologist, and explained what was happening. They said, 'That's OK. Call us when you're ready.' "I cleared the room, moved the bed over, got a tape deck. The man and his wife put on their wedding music, and they danced. All of us nurses outside the door were crying our eyes out. It was beautiful, and it happened because of a team effort, and care for the patient. 'That's OK. Call us when you're ready.' How amazing is that!"

Marjorie Wiggins encapsulated all this quite succinctly: "It's the nurturing part of nursing that we all love."

Brenda Zimmerman, PhD, CA, MBA, BSc, is professor of strategic management at Schulich School of Business, York University, Toronto. She is the founder and director of the Health Industry Management Program for MBA students. Her volunteer commitments in healthcare include service on the Science Advisory Board of Plexus Institute, membership on an advisory committee of the Canadian Royal College of Physicians and Surgeons, service as an advisor to the Canadian Public Health Agency; and membership on the Board of Mount Sinai Hospital in Toronto. Her latest co-authored book, *Getting to Maybe: How the World is Changed* is a Canadian best seller. She is also co-author of *Edgeware: Insights from Complexity Science for Health Care Leaders.*

San Ng, MBA, BSc, is principal and founder of Vision & Results Inc., a healthcare management consulting firm. San has extensive experience consulting across the healthcare sector including the Ministry of Health and Long-Term Care and Ministry of Community and Social Services. San is currently completing a PhD in organization management in the Department of Health Policy, Management and Evaluation at the University of Toronto. She holds an MBA from McMaster University. San is Past Chair of the Canadian College of Health Service Executives, Greater Toronto Area Chapter and previous Board Member of Responsible Gambling Ontario and the Canadian Association of Management Consultants.

Works Cited

1. F. Wald and A. Toynbee, The Hospice Experiment, 2007.

2. C. F. von Gunten and T. Ryndes, "The Academic Hospice," *Annals of Internal Medicine* 143, no. 9 (2005): 655-658.

3. R. Stacey, *Complex Responsive Processes in Organizations: Learning and Knowledge Creation* (London: Routledge, 2001).

4. R. D. Stacey, D. Griffin, and P. Shaw, *Complexity and Management: Fad or Radical Challenge to Systems Thinking* (London: Routledge, 2000).

5. P. Zurn, C. Dolea, and B. Stilwell, "Issue 4: Nurse Retention and Recruitment: Developing a Motivated Workforce," *The Global Nursing Review Initiative: World Health Organization, Department of Human Resources for Health* (2005).

6. H. Dershin, "Nonlinear Systems Theory in Medical Care Management," *Physician Executive* 25, no. 3 (1999): 8-13.

7. R. L. Hoffman, "The Evolution of Hospice in America: Nursing's Role in the Movement," *Journal of Gerontology and Nursing* 31 (2005): 26-34, 30.

8. D. Cooperrider, "Positive Image, Positive Action: The Affirmative Basis of Organizing," in *Appreciative Management and Leadership: The Power of Positive Thought and Action in Organizations*, ed. S. Sirvastva and D. L. Cooperider. (San Francisco: Josse-Bass, 1990), 91-125.

9. D. Cooperrider and S. Srivastva, "Appreciative Inquiry in Organizational Life," *Research in Organizational Change and Development* 1 (1987): 129-169.

10. G. Bushe, "Advances in Appreciative Inquiry As an Organizational Development Intervention," *Organizational Development Journal* 13, no. 3 (1995): 14-22.

11. G. Russell and J. Fawcett, "A Conceptual Model of Nursing and Health Policy," *Policy, Politics and Nursing Practice* 2, no. 2 (2001): 108-116.

12. G. Russell and J. Fawcett, "The Conceptual Model for Nursing and Health Policy Revisited," *Policy, Politics and Nursing Practice* 6, no. 4 (2005): 319-326.

13. C. H. Ellenbecker, J. Fawcett, and G. Glazer, "A Nursing PhD Specialty in Health Policy: University of Massachusetts Boston," *Policy, Politics and Nursing Practice* 6 (2005): 229-235.

14. L. Abdallah, "EverCare Nurse Practitioner Practice Activities: Similarities and Differences Across Five Sites" (Doctoral Dissertation, University of Massachusetts, 2003).

15. L. Cestari-Long, "Impact of Medicare Payment Policies for Home Healthcare on Nursing Services and Patient Outcomes" (Doctoral Dissertation, University of Massachusetts, 2005).

16. K. Donaher, "The Human Capital Competencies Inventory for Nurse Managers: Development and Psychometric Testing" (Doctoral Dissertation, University of Massachusetts, 2004).

17. S. A. LaRocco, "Policies and Practices that Influence Recruitment and Retention of Men in Nursing: A Grounded Theory Study of Socializing Men" (Doctoral Dissertation, University of Massachusetts, 2004).

18. E. O'Connell, "Considering the Alternatives: The White House Commission on Complementary and Alternative Medicine Study" (Doctoral Dissertation, University of Massachusetts, 2002).

19. P. A. Poirier, "The Relation of Sick Leave Benefits, Employment Patterns, and Individual Characteristics to Radiation Therapy-related Fatigue" (Doctoral Dissertation, University of Massachusetts, 2005).

20. A. W. Lochler and J. Didion, "Epidemic to Endemic: The Impact of HIV on Healthcare Policy and Nursing Practice," *Policy, Politics and Nursing Practice* 4, no. 1 (2003): 62-70.

21. UNAIDS and WHO, "AIDS Epidemic Update: Special Report on HIV/AIDS," 2008. Available from http://www.unaids.org/en/KnowledgeCentre/HIVData/EpiUpdate/EpiUp-dArchive/2006/Default.asp.

22. P. W. Stone et al., "Evidence of Nurse Working Conditions: A Global Perspective," *Policy, Politics and Nursing Practice* 4, no. 2 (2003): 120-130.

23. D. D. Affonso and D. Doran, "Cultivating Discoveries in Patient Safety Research: A Framework," *International Journal of Nursing Perspectives* 2, no. 1 (2002): 33-47.

24. American Hospital Association, "Pathways for Medication Safety," 2008. Available from www.medpathways.info.

25. Lewin, R., and B. Regine, "Where's the Care," 2008. Available from http://www.plexusinstitute.org/ideas/show_story.cfm?id=29.

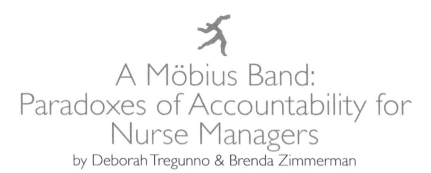

A Möbius Band:
Paradoxes of Accountability for Nurse Managers

by Deborah Tregunno & Brenda Zimmerman

A mathematician confided
That a Möbius band is one-sided,
And you'll get quite a laugh,
If you cut one in half,
For it stays in one piece when divided[1]

In everyday conversations, paradox and contradiction are often treated as synonyms. Yet they are not the same. Two opposites that cannot co-exist make a contradiction. Both sides cannot be true at the same time. Yet a paradox, like the Möbius band, is when apparent opposites co-exist. Both sides are simultaneously true. We believe nurse managers are facing paradoxes in accountability which, when treated in traditional evaluation frameworks as contradictions, inadvertently impede true accountability. In this chapter, we will explore three paradoxes and how to approach them with a Complexity Science perspective in mind.

Severe Acute Respiratory Syndrome (SARS) in Toronto, Ontario

On Saturday April 5, 2004, André Picard, the public health reporter for *The Globe And* Mail, Canada's national newspaper,[2] filed this story on a mysterious killer that was playing havoc in Toronto, Ontario:

> It was a routine patient transfer. Mount Sinai Hospital in downtown Toronto is renowned for fighting infectious diseases, so troublesome cases often wind up there. On this Sunday night, the ambulance brought a patient from Scarborough Hospital, who was suffering from severe respiratory problems. A nurse in intensive care greeted the ambulance and helped the patient settle in. The man coughed, and coughed. He burned with fever. She bathed him with soothing cold water and offered comforting words. "I've had a lot of patients with atypical pneumonia over the years," the nurse said. "This wasn't that different. I just did my job, caring for the patient as best I could."

> But this was different. The man had severe acute respiratory syndrome (SARS), and the Monday-morning papers would reveal he was the 13th patient in an increasingly worrisome outbreak. As she did her work, the nurse took respiratory precautions, wearing a mask, gloves and a gown. But there was a period of time, during the transfer, when the nurse was unprotected, breathing in a potentially deadly virus. By Wednesday morning, the hospital had called to say she was under quarantine, and to monitor herself for SARS symptoms: a fever over 38 degrees Celsius, a dry cough, and difficulty breathing. After taking her temperature, she checked herself into the hospital, where her workplace, the intensive-care unit, became her prison.[2]

Managing the SARS outbreak was arguably one of the most complicated and confusing challenges ever faced by Ontario's healthcare managers, and it was laden with paradoxes. *Care for patients! Keep nurses safe!*
The main locus of transmission was hospitals, where forty-five percent of
the people who contracted the illness were healthcare workers. *Keep beds
open. Be efficient!* The outbreak highlighted existing human resource issues, such as nursing shortages, workforce casualization (temporary staff),
and the everyday workplace dangers of violence, abuse, exposure to toxic
chemicals, bodily fluids, and infectious diseases. *Manage the situation! Stay
on budget!* The economic toll was devastating. Hospital budgets soared out
of control with added overtime and infection control costs. In the wider
community, conventions and bus tours were cancelled, with the cancella-
tion of 1.3 million trips from the United States to Canada in the spring
months of 2003.[3] By July 2003, when Ontario's public health officials de-
clared that the SARS epidemic was over, it had killed a total of forty-four
people in Toronto, Ontario including two nurses and a doctor. *Be innovative! Predict the future!*

According to Picard,[2] the first person to spot SARS in Toronto was a
nurse manager at Scarborough Hospital:

> It was the weekend, so Agnes Wang spent a little time
> scanning the Chinese-language papers. She's a nurse and
> one story caught her eye: a father and daughter who had
> died from a strange form of pneumonia that had popped
> up in Hong Kong. When she got to work on Monday
> morning, Ms. Wang, began to review charts. She was
> struck by the fact that one patient, 44-year-old Toronto res-
> ident, Mr. Tse, had a strange breed of pneumonia, and his
> mother had died a few days earlier, also suffering from a
> mysterious respiratory ailment. "I said: 'This is a strange
> coincidence.' And I asked one of the nurses to check the
> patient's travel history," Ms. Wang recalled. "It turns out
> his mother had visited Hong Kong." The night before, in-
> fection-control officers had been notified, as they are
> whenever there is an unusual pathogen. But Ms. Wang's

observation allowed public-health investigators to connect the dots. And so began the detective work related to Canada's outbreak of severe acute respiratory syndrome (SARS). Ms. Wang said it is nice to know she played a part in helping stem the outbreak, but she gives much of the credit to colleague Sandy Finkelstein. As director of the intensive-care unit, he had placed Mr. Tse in isolation, on a hunch. Dr. Finkelstein, in turn, credits the nurse for her sharp eye. Either way, the double dose of serendipity probably limited the spread of SARS dramatically.

Within days, at least seven people who came into contact with Mr. Tse, directly or indirectly, died. Dozens of others became ill and, because of the rippling web of contacts, hundreds more under quarantine. However, had the gravely ill patient not been isolated and the connection to Hong Kong not made so soon, many more nurses would have had direct contact with Mr. Tse. "What's happening is pretty bad," Ms. Wang said, "but it could have been much, much worse. Sure, if we had known ahead of time what we were dealing with, we could have done more. . . . But it turns out we were actually very lucky."[2]

Did the SARS situation place unique demands on nurse managers? Although the SARS situation was extraordinary, in this chapter we suggest that by the very nature of their role, nurses in management positions face complex challenges daily. Nurse managers care for individuals, families, and communities by working with nurses and other healthcare professionals to provide care that produces optimal outcomes. Through the formal authority conferred on them, nurse managers are given the responsibility to accomplish specific goals for the organization, and are held accountable for their performance.

Accountability is understood as the obligation to answer for a responsibility that has been conferred. This implies a formal relationship in which one person acts as the agent for another. By the virtue of their position and authority, nurse managers are agents for many stakeholders who can have competing interests and expectations of the managers' role and actions. For example, the SARS situation required managers *to keep staff safe* and *to care for patients*. At first glance, this requirement seems to defy intuition. Caring for patients often requires an intimacy, a close physical proximity, and providing time for the patient with close family and friends to aid with the healing process. Yet to be safe, staff needed to be physically distant from these patients. Are nurse managers accountable for both of these responsibilities at the same time, in the same practice setting? In this chapter, we explore this question by examining the paradox of accountability for nurse managers, and offer students of nursing management and leadership new ways to see and respond to seemingly contradictory demands. This paper addresses three questions:

> *We have identified three areas of tension for nurse managers in today's demanding practice settings: 1) efficiency and effectiveness, 2) task and relationship, and 3) stability and change.*

- What paradoxes of nursing management exist in healthcare practice settings?

- How does a complexity-inspired approach to nursing management differ from traditional practice?

- How can Complexity Science help nurse managers improve outcomes of care?

Paradoxes of Nursing Management

We have identified three areas of tension for nurse managers in today's demanding practice settings: 1) efficiency and effectiveness, 2) task and relationship, and 3) stability and change. Any of these can pose seemingly contradictory responsibilities for nurse managers in their daily activities. Each is explored below.

Efficiency and Effectiveness

The Institute of Medicine's publication *Crossing the Quality Chasm*[4] calls for improvement in six dimensions of healthcare performance: safety, patient-centeredness, timeliness, equity, effectiveness, and efficiency. Although all six dimensions are important, in this section we will focus on the tension between effectiveness and efficiency.

The Institute of Medicine defines efficiency as the avoidance of waste, including waste of equipment, ideas, and energy. The call for improved efficiency asks nurse managers to look at the relationship between resource inputs and clinical outputs. "Do more with less" is the de facto expectation.

Nurse managers are accountable for the presence of adequate, qualified, and competent staff who will provide quality nursing care. Because nurses are the primary providers of patient care and account for the largest portion of the labor budget in many healthcare organizations, adjustments to staffing levels and skill mix are some of the key ways for nurse managers to manipulate resource inputs. Accordingly, nurse managers face challenging decisions about appropriate staffing levels, skill mix,[5;6] and care delivery models.[7] In addition, nurse managers make decisions about the practice environment that influence the efficiency with which nurses and other healthcare professionals carry out their work, including factors such as the communication systems, the physical layout,[8] the availability and use of information technology,[9] the nursing team composition, and the work environment,[10-12] and overtime hours.[13] In response to questions of appropriate nurse staffing and patient safety, some governmental jurisdictions have already regulated staffing levels while others are considering legislation in this area.[14] Others call for increased attention to performance measurement of nursing care in order to demonstrate nurses' contribution to patient outcomes.[15;16]

At the same time, nurse managers are also focused on effectiveness, which is defined by the Institute of Medicine[4] as the provision of services based on scientific knowledge and the avoidance of services not likely to benefit the patient. The rise of evidence-based practice is seen as a response to long-term efforts to close the gap between research and practice, and as a way to hold healthcare practitioners accountable for the quality and cost of healthcare.[17;18] Evidence-based practice is a problem solving approach that integrates the best available scientific evidence, nurses' clinical expertise, and patients' preferences and values.[19] Described as a way for nurses to establish their professional role in relation to patient outcomes,[20] there are indications that the implementation of evidence-based practice improves the cost-effectiveness of patient care.[21-24] In addition, managers are accountable for ensuring compliance with professional and regulatory standards of care and scope of practice.

Despite the benefits of evidence-based practice, there are many barriers to nurses' use of research in everyday practice.[25;26] Strategies for advancing evidence-based practice in clinical practice settings often focus on the need for shared knowledge about the evidence and how to incorporate evidence into practice, clinical champions, and technological infrastructure for guideline dissemination and monitoring of use, time, and money.[27]

A paradox looms: For a clinical practice setting to run efficiently, a balance must be struck between nurse inputs and the delivery of effective patient care. At the same time, evidence-based practice cannot be implemented or sustained without appropriate nursing inputs. How do nurse managers balance the competing demands of efficiency and effectiveness given the inextricable link between these two demands?

Task and Relationship

The second paradox of accountability is the tension between task orientation and relationship management.

To be task oriented, nurse managers must draw on knowledge and competencies in many areas. These include technical and procedural skills, and knowledge of the physiology and pharmacology of health and illness. Timing of interventions—including meals, drugs, and visitors, in addition to turn-around times for tests and procedures—need to be monitored to ensure the tasks of caring for the patient are accomplished.

However, nurse managers also need to address the relationship aspects of care. These include patient-provider relationships and interprofessional relationships as well as the social and political aspects that influence day-to-day life of patients and coworkers. There are issues of teamwork and interprofessional collaboration. These things shape how nurses make sense of their context, and how they choose to enact their values in professional practice.

Task and relationship are often viewed as different kinds of approaches to nursing situations. Task orientation often involves specific guidelines and protocols to follow, with standardization being seen as a virtue. Accountability is interpreted as adherence to the appropriate guideline and plan of care. Explicit knowledge is highly valued and documentation is key. On the other hand, tacit knowledge is a key in relationship management. Rather than standardization, extreme customization is required as each relationship is unique. Every relationship requires the nurse manager to be highly cognizant of context and to respond, often with little documented guidance, but rather based on a strong sense of values and broad parameters or principles of professional practice. Accountability in this case would need to take into consideration the specific circumstances faced.

In the midst of the current nursing shortage, it is increasingly important for nurse managers to understand the nature of nursing practice behaviors. Many hospital nurses perform isolated and routine task-centered care, which is viewed as analogous to the diagnostic approach to healthcare. An assumption of this approach to patient care is that the nurse, or expert, defines and performs or delegates the definitive interventions to control and manage the patient's health. Some authors suggest that the diagnostic approach allows nurses to label the clients' conditions in relation to nursing assessments, a normative set of problems, and expected outcomes.[28] As the expert, the nurse discovers and responds to the patient's objective reality in a manner similar to the way physicians make a diagnosis and treatment plan. This standardized approach to patient assessment is seen as a way to achieve greater professional accountability by moving nurses to an outcome focus and towards monitoring and evaluating the efficiency and effectiveness of the care they provide.[29]

Others argue that the hallmarks of professional nursing practice are relationships and the delivery of individualized patient care that reflects the dignity and value of all persons as individuals. An assumption of the individualized approach to care is that nurses need to spend time with the patient, get to know the patient, and develop responsive relationships built on respect, trust, and mutuality.[30] For individualized care, nurses combine this patient knowledge with scientific knowledge to select optimal therapeutic interventions.[31] Through development of responsive relationships, patient-centered clinical decisions are guided by integrating knowledge of the patient's preferences, practices, and capabilities with the best available evidence.

A paradox looms: Nurse managers are responsible for supervision of other nurses and are accountable for quality of care delivered to patients and families. Task-oriented and relationship-focused care are often viewed as two distinct approaches to nursing practice. How do nurse managers make sense of the tension between task-oriented and relationship-focused care?

Change and Continuity

The third paradox relates to change and stability or continuity: to innovate and adapt and yet to keep things on track and predictable.

Today's nursing practice environment is continually undergoing significant changes. Balanced budgets, performance measurement, benchmarking, cultural diversity, quality management, multidisciplinary teams, downsizing, capitated systems, and nursing shortages, are but a few examples of the changes which nurse managers must respond to. In addition, nursing is impacted by demographic changes such as homelessness, unemployment, increased numbers of uninsured and under-insured, the growing elderly population, and increased globalization. Successful change depends on a process that is hard to manage and involves multiple stakeholders who take on different roles at different stages in the implementation process.[32] The world around us is changing, and nurse managers play an important role in determining what the future can bring and what it will be like for patients and families as well as healthcare providers.

How do nurse managers make sense of the tension between task-oriented and relationship-focused care?

Much has been written to assist nurse managers with change. At the individual level, staged theories have been offered to describe a path to action. Much of this work is rooted in the theory of reasoned action[33] and suggests that individuals pass through a series of stages as they approach a new behavior. For instance, the awareness-to-adherence model, which outlines the steps to compliance with the use of clinical practice guidelines,[34] suggests that compliance with practice guidelines requires passage through four stages: (1) become aware of the guidelines, (2) intellectually agree with them, (3) decide to adopt them, and finally, (4) regularly adhere to the guidelines as indicated. Even though this type of model leaves little hope for change among those who "fall off the path," this approach to change suggests that nurse managers can address behavior changes only after they attend to issues of awareness and attitude.

At the level of the organization, change models[35;36] can help nurse managers understand changes in relation to the practice environment. Given the importance of context, it is not surprising that Gustafson et al.[35] found that flexibility, or the degree to which the change design fits into existing context, is predictive of successful change. The climate of the work environment, including well-defined reporting relationships[37] and staff incentives[38] has also been shown to influence the success of change initiatives. A simple implementation plan, complete with carefully defined roles, responsibilities, a schedule, and feedback, also increases the likelihood of successful change.[39]

The other side of the paradox is continuity and stability. Nurse managers are held responsible for keeping their units predictable and on track, in addition to maintaining the status quo. Predictability can play a role in improving care. For example, in the patient safety movement, stability in the team can lead to a comfort with interprofessional relationships and the ability to understand what colleagues expect and need to perform at their best.[40]

Everything cannot change all of the time. At an individual level, nurses interested in continuity and stability may feel the need to reduce uncertainty associated with the change all around them. Some nurses may be focused on continuity so that they can maintain a coherent self-concept, which may not be possible in a practice environment that challenges them to reflect on core values and assumptions that may differ from those they developed in their professional training. Moreover, there are individual differences in preferences for stability and change, including tolerance for ambiguity and openness to experience.[41] Some nurses, and nurse managers, are just better able to tolerate change than others.

A paradox looms: The current emphasis on change in our healthcare environment fails to recognize that change and stability complement each other and are simultaneous forces affecting individuals and organizational actions. How do nurse managers respond to the push and pull of change and continuity? How do they mobilize energy for change while managing continuity?

Other chapters in this book define Complexity Science and provide numerous examples of complexity principles applied to nursing. In this chapter, we will draw on these concepts and principles, applying them to evaluation and accountability frameworks. But first we will return to the story of SARS to look at how complexity played out in practice.

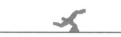

A paradox looms: The current emphasis on change in our healthcare environment fails to recognize that change and stability complement each other and are simultaneous forces affecting individuals and organizational actions.

SARS – In Vancouver, British Colombia

Vancouver's SARS response took a dramatically different path. The province of British Columbia (BC) avoided the major outbreak of SARS experienced in Ontario, where most of the cases resulted from hospital-based exposure. Three of five international importations of SARS to Canada came through Vancouver, but they were spread to only one other person. In total, there were just four probable cases of SARS in BC and no deaths.

British Columbia's good fortune has been largely attributed to numerous alerts issued by the British Columbia Centre for Disease Control, warning of an imminent threat from Asia. Vancouver General Hospital was in a state of readiness and nurses responded by masking patient zero within minutes of arrival at the emergency room and by maintaining a heightened level of infection control. By notifying the BC Centre for Disease Control, Vancouver General Hospital helped put the world on alert that SARS had spread beyond Southeast Asia and was a global threat. "Simply put," says Dr. Danuta Skowronski, Epidemiologist, BC Centre for Disease Control, "British Columbians owe the clinicians and staff of Vancouver General Hospital a collective debt of gratitude. They have shown that in the battle against infectious disease, a combination of vigilance, infection control and good communication can be very effective."[42]

Dr. Skowronski has argued that BC was successful in limiting the spread of SARS for two reasons. First, the province-wide system of infection control and alerts was effective. Second, BC was "lucky" that the first SARS patient was admitted to Vancouver General Hospital, which had excellent internal infection control systems, good communication within the hospital and, in short, was well-managed. This is "lucky" for the government because it can't directly control the way a hospital is managed. But it is not luck at the hospital level. Indeed, it is the job of a hospital's leaders.[42]

Three separate awards were given at the Annual Appreciation Dinner hosted by the British Columbia Centre for Disease Control on Friday, November 28, 2003. Awards recognized the excellence of staff of the Emergency Department, the Intensive Care Unit, and the Medical Microbiology and Infection Control Division at Vancouver General Hospital. The awards recognized staff for being exceptionally alert and responsive in the early stages of an emerging respiratory threat.

> Front-line public health and clinical staff across British Columbia have much to be proud of in responding to SARS, says Dr. Perry Kendall, Provincial Health Officer. Together, they prevented British Columbians from suffering a severe respiratory outbreak. We are giving special recognition to Vancouver General Hospital because it demonstrated a terrific level of baseline preparedness and infection control before SARS was even recognized as a global threat.[43]

What lessons are there in this story to address the paradoxes of accountability: 1) efficiency and effectiveness, 2) task and relationship, and 3) stability and change? What role does evaluation—formal and informal—play in addressing these paradoxes?

Accountability and Evaluation Frameworks

In *Getting to Maybe*, Westley, Zimmerman, and Patton[44] explore two evaluation paradigms related to social innovation and change: summative and developmental. A summary of the key differences between these approaches is provided in Table 1.

As illustrated in Table 1, summative evaluations are typically rational and goal-directed, and see performance as a linear relationship between inputs, processes, and outputs. Goals are clearly defined, performance measures are pre-determined, data collection protocols are rigid, and the standards against which goal achievement is assessed are externally established. Evaluators who adopt the summative paradigm tend to use carefully developed protocols and procedures to ensure a standardized approach to data collection and analysis. Accountability is focused on compliance with prescribed and approved procedures and goal attainment.

Summative evaluations are ideal for one side of the paradoxes: efficiency, task, and stability. Logic models are designed with a clear sense of

Table 1: Summative and Developmental Approach to Evaluation

Summative Evaluation	Developmental Evaluation
Render definitive judgments of success or failure	Provide feedback, generate learning, support changes in direction
Traditional, linear, using step by step logic model that outlines inputs, activities, and processes required to achieve expected outcomes	Complexity-informed, fluid, ambiguous, ever changing, joining inquiry and action, openness to what emerges is the goal while moving toward an envisioned future
Accountability focused on and directed to external authorities and stakeholders	Accountability centered on the innovator's deep sense of fundamental values and commitment
Accountability to control and locate responsibility	Learning to respond to lack of control and stay in touch with what's unfolding and thereby respond strategically
Measure success against predetermined goals	Develop new measures and monitoring mechanisms as goals emerge and evolve
Learning is about how to attain desired outcomes	Learning is about the appropriateness of the intended outcomes in relation to emergent opportunities
Evaluation separated from innovation, or that which is being assessed	Evaluation is integral to those bringing about the change
Success or failure based on goal attainment; little or no attention to unanticipated outcomes	Success is based on openness to what emerges against backdrop of changing goals; unanticipated outcomes provide an opportunity for corrective action
Accountability focuses on compliance with prescribed and approved procedures and attaining intended results	Accountability focuses on learning that will inform future action

the input and output relationships. Hence, efficiency can be improved by tracking performance against these predetermined goals and input-output connections. It is ideally designed for task evaluation as one can prescribe expected behaviors or procedures and assess compliance against these standards. Since goals, outcomes, and procedures are prescribed a priori it is well suited for maintaining patterns, in other words for stability.

The balanced scorecard approach reflects a traditional accountability framework, or summative perspective on evaluation. Developed by Kaplan and Norton[45] and used by business and healthcare organizations, the balanced scorecard provides a framework to translate strategic objectives and goals into a coherent, balanced, and multidimensional set of performance measures that help monitor the trade-offs between strategic and operational decisions. Accordingly, the scorecard tells the story of the strategy, starting with the long-run financial objectives, and then linking them to the sequence of actions that must be taken with financial processes, customers, internal processes, and finally employees and systems to deliver the desired long-run economic performance. The balanced scorecard dimensions of performance, which include internal business process, financial, learning and growth, and customer, are described in Table 2.

Information on efficiency, tasks, and stability—which are arguably more straightforward to address within the traditional accountability framework—is accounted for in the balanced scorecard format. For instance, balanced scorecards in healthcare include data on clinical productivity and efficiency,[46] access to care,[47] quality and customer satisfaction,[48]

Table 2: The Balanced Scorecard Dimensions of Performance

Internal Business Process	Financial	Learning & Growth	Customer
Emphasizes internal processes to achieve customer expectations and financial goals (including quality, response time, cost, and new product introductions).	Emphasizes return on investment and economic value added; achievement of shareholder objectives.	Emphasis on infrastructure to enable achievement of the objectives in other three domains (including employee capabilities and information systems capabilities).	Emphasizes alignment of core customer outcome measures (satisfaction, retention, and profitability) to financial objectives.

and finances.[49] Performance is evaluated using a limited number of indicators which are selected to show the achievement of success.[50] While developed mainly at the executive level, nurse managers use scorecard data for accountability in two important ways. First, because nurse managers operate at the interface between senior management and the clinicians who deliver care, they play a critical role in communicating and operationalizing the organization's strategic directions. The balanced scorecard facilitates managers' decision making and provides a structure to communicate strategic goals and objectives to all staff.[49] The second way that the balanced scorecard framework helps nurse managers is by providing a set of indicators that demonstrates the complex, interdependent, and potentially paradoxical nature of workflow. For example, nurse managers can use scorecard data to interpret the link between financial measures of efficiency (task measures) such as staffing costs, and internal processes such as turnaround times for diagnostic procedures in the emergency department.[51]

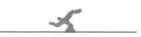

In the real world of nurse managers, as exemplified by the SARS story, unpredictability abounds and accountability needs to incorporate the ability to respond to unanticipated contexts.

Summative evaluation has some glaring weaknesses, however, when we are dealing with the other side of the paradoxes—effectiveness, relationship, and change—and indeed with paradox in general. Summative evaluations need clarity and hence ambiguity is often ignored. Unanticipated outcomes—emergence—are also not evaluated. Hence the accountability framework implicit in the summative evaluation mode is one in which nurse managers should know a priori what is expected and learning is limited to attaining predetermined outcomes. In the real world of nurse managers, as exemplified by the SARS story, unpredictability abounds and accountability needs to incorporate the ability to respond to unanticipated contexts.

On the other side of the paradoxes, one could argue that questions of effectiveness, relationship, and change need something beyond traditional frameworks. They are harder to nail down in formulae or standardized expectations. When we look at these as paradoxes rather than either-or choices, traditional frames are clearly inadequate to the task. Complexity

Science offers some insights into how to complement traditional accountability frameworks with evaluation approaches that embrace effectiveness, relationships, and change.

Based on Michael Patton's work on developmental evaluation, Westley, Zimmerman and Patton[44] offer the developmental paradigm as a complexity-informed approach to evaluation. It is designed to address contexts where problems are not bounded, do not have optimal solutions, and do not occur within stable parameters. See Table 1. According to Gamble, evaluation is related to critical thinking and development is related to creative thinking. These two types of thinking are often considered to be mutually exclusive. Gamble proposes that developmental evaluation is holds them both in balance.[52]

From a developmental perspective, evaluators focus on short-term desired outcomes *and* on longer-term opportunities that emerge over time. Developmental evaluations demand attention to what emerges as possibility, and assessment of the degree to which the intended outcomes are appropriate in the given situation. Success and/or failure in the developmental paradigm are judged in relation to learning about what is and is not working. Inquiry is closely linked with action and approaches to data collection change over time to correspond to the ebb and flow of information. From the complexity perspective, accountability focuses on the use of feedback to devise opportunities for future improvement. Accountability focuses on learning that will inform future action. A key component of this learning is the ability to respond to lack of control and stay in touch with what is emerging. By being very attentive to the patterns that are arising and by continuing to be open to new data, unanticipated outcomes can provide important information for new actions. In essence, the measure against which comparisons are made are not predetermined outcomes, but values—commitments to broad missions and mandates. The focus is on effectiveness more than efficiency. Ensuring the right things are being done is crucial.

Relationships are vital in developmental evaluation and are important to help make sense of emerging patterns. Connectedness of the players across the organization and between organizations is crucial to ensure that information flows swiftly and effectively to those who can act upon it. In addition, personal relationships are needed to ensure the whole team or system is paying attention and players at all levels are being heard. In addition, relationships are an important part of accountability as developmental evaluation depends on preparation for unanticipated patterns. Nurse managers can act as key role models and leaders in demonstrating, teaching, and expecting their teams to ask questions that will enhance everyone's capacity to recognize and respond to emergence in an effective

Table 3: Developmental evaluation sample of techniques
(Adapted from Gamble, 2007)

What? So what? Now what? Basic heuristic to analyze multiple factors in the moment and to align diverse actions toward common interests.
Examples:
What? What do we see? What does data tell us? What are the indicators of change or stability? How can we capture changing patterns as they emerge?

So what? So, what sense can we make of emerging data? What does it mean to us in this moment and in the future? What effect is this likely to have on our patients, colleagues, and our extended network?

Now what? What are our options? When and how can we act—individually and collectively—to optimize opportunities in this moment and the next? How and to whom can we communicate? How can we ensure what is seen locally, regionally, and globally is being spread across the network in an effective manner? What is our role in improving this?

Network mapping. Mapping a network is a process of identifying connections between people and graphically displaying those connections.
Example:
Tracking how ideas are shared and spread and where participants take joint action can indicate where natural strengths exist and also where there are weaknesses in the network.

Appreciative Inquiry. This is a mode of inquiry originated by David Cooperrider which asks what is working and why it is effective.
Example:
By asking appreciative inquiry questions, behaviors that are effective at recognizing patterns and or relationships that are effective at spreading information can surface and be used deliberately to improve effectiveness.

Simulations. In a complex environment, we ask questions about different change conditions. This can be done as a mental exercise individually or with a team. Or it can be assisted with computer software.
Example:
Ask questions such as: What will happen if we change this? Or that? The idea is to simulate a variety of contexts to increase the capacity to see emerging patterns and to respond quickly and effectively.

manner. Table 3 provides some examples of developmental evaluation techniques.

Cook and Rasmussen[53] provide a complexity-informed model of system dynamics that is consistent with the developmental approach to evaluation. In the "going solid"* model of system dynamics, Cook and Rasmussen focus on nature of the operating space, defined as an envelope created by economic, workload, and performance boundaries. Because the environment is dynamic, the location of the operating point is influenced by tensions between workload and economic failure. Changes in the gradients can move the operating point toward the unacceptable performance boundary. The model presented in Figure 1, which is adapted from Cook and Rasmussen illustrates two operating points. A safe operating space, as represented by point "A," occurs when the tension between economic and workload demands is balanced so that the operating space is contained within the boundaries of economic efficiency, workload, and performance. When economic and workload tensions are not balanced, changes in the gradients will cause a shift in the operating space across the boundary of optimal performance to an unsafe space, as illustrated in Figure 1 by point "B." Cook and Rasmussen suggest that the operating system is "going solid" when the safe space moves across the boundary of acceptable performance. Further, Cook and Rasmussen remind us that the boundary of

Figure 1: System dynamics of safe operating space

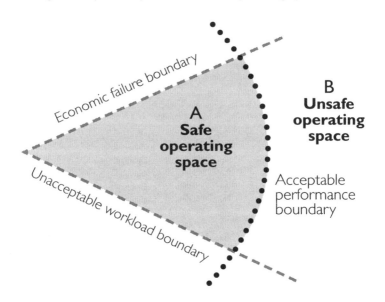

acceptable performance is unknown, and that only violations of practice standards provide information about its position.

Healthcare often operates at the margin of acceptable performance in order to minimize economic costs and workload. Moreover, nurse managers are painfully aware of how their units are often working at the limit of their capacity, and of how seemingly small changes can send the unit to the margins of acceptable performance.

SARS – The Different Paths in Toronto and Vancouver

Vancouver, British Colombia did better in its response to SARS than Toronto, Ontario. Vancouver had more robust and collaborative worker safety, infection control, and public health systems than Toronto, which contributed to BC's better containment of the index case. In contrast, Toronto experienced poor communication, and unlike their colleagues in BC, healthcare workers across Ontario were not alerted to the emergence of a new disease in China and Hong Kong.

Considering the differences between the Toronto and Vancouver SARS response, Farjoun and Zimmerman[42] look forward to what hospitals can do to fight the next SARS-like crisis. Recalling that organizations, particularly those dealing with high-risk tasks, are prone to accidents, Farjoun and Zimmerman remind us that some are better prepared and more resilient than others. Some accidents may happen because of operator errors, others because of inappropriate organizational arrangements and flawed decision making, and yet others because of broader causes at the policy and societal levels. Often accidents happen because of multiple factors across different levels. Reports from the 9/11 Commission and the Columbia Accident Investigation Board, for example, have stressed understanding the organizational level—the way organizations operate, their structure and processes, culture, and managerial practices—because this often holds a critical key to better diagnosis and prognosis. Moreover, the actual behavior of dedicated and well-intentioned healthcare workers is heavily influ-

---

* In nuclear energy generation, management of the steam boiler requires the presence of both steam and water. When the boiler becomes full of water, because of a change in temperature, the resulting situation is hazardous and difficult to manage. This is referred to as "going solid." For more information on water coolant systems, please refer to

enced by their local team environment, organizational routines and practices, policy and management decisions, organizational culture, and professional and occupational norms. Although there were many heroes in the SARS story, effectively managed hospitals should produce consistent results independent of particular individuals.

Accountability for nurse managers needs to incorporate the concept of resilience and the ability to respond in high-risk situations. In reviewing the stories of Vancouver's and Toronto's approaches to SARS, it is interesting to review the techniques listed on Table 3. In both cases, front-line nurses were first to recognize the threat. But in BC, this recognition very quickly spread up, down, and across the system. In Vancouver, the system was robust and resilient because the work had been done in advance to ensure that information could spread easily across the system from the front line to the hospital risk team and to the province and information from the global level was also effectively connected to the region and local players. The network was relationship-rich and created the conditions for quick and effective sharing of patterns as they emerged. In Vancouver, the basic heuristic of what, so what, and now what was widely shared throughout the system. Local knowledge and learning was respected and acted upon. The Vancouver response indicated an awareness of resilience and a capacity to act on unanticipated outcomes.

Accountability for nurse managers needs to incorporate the concept of resilience and the ability to respond in high-risk situations.

In Toronto, although a nurse manager noted the first case of SARS and was instrumental in stemming the tide of the disease, the system was not nearly as effective as in Vancouver. Barriers in communication in the Toronto, Ontario networks meant that patterns that reoccurred in other hospitals were not recognized, and hence the same high-risk behaviors that created the first deaths of patients and healthcare providers were repeated in a second wave of the infection. In addition, nurses in some hospitals found that although they saw the patterns, there was no effective way for them to share the information upward and across in the system. Many nurses decried the lack of respect for their locally derived knowledge and pattern recognition, and claimed this led to many unnecessary infections and deaths. The system in Toronto and Ontario relied on hierarchy, in a top-down fashion, to sense the patterns and make decisions. This slowed down response time and also created a separation of local and macro knowledge. Learning did happen, but it was hampered by a system which paid little heed to the local organizational factors, such as culture, and their links to public policy.

Complexity – The Different Path for Nurse Managers

To be truly accountable at the highest and most appropriate level for healthcare, nurse managers need to accept paradox as normal and embrace approaches which allow them to be accountable for the full range of their responsibilities.

In considering how a complexity lens moves nurse managers to fuller accountability, it is helpful to reconsider the difference between the Toronto and Vancouver SARS experiences in light of Cook and Rasmussen's model of system dynamics. At the outset of the Toronto experience, standard operating procedures were in use. The goal was to provide the most appropriate care to individual patients who presented to emergency departments. From a summative perspective, goal achievement was focused on balancing competing patient demands and delivery of patient care. SARS patients were transferred between organizations to receive specialized care. Respiratory precautions, which increase workload, were not taken by nurses and doctors. On the whole, healthcare providers and managers were not aware that the emerging situation was moving the operating point beyond the acceptable boundary of performance. Simply stated, healthcare providers did not know that the system was "going solid" and that they were operating in an unsafe space. As stated earlier in the chapter, serendipity played a major role in limiting the spread of SARS in Toronto.

In contrast, the early warnings of an imminent threat from Asia alerted Vancouver's healthcare providers to be on the lookout for the global threat. In addition to providing standard emergency department care to their patients, they were attentive to the emergent situation. By all accounts, they were vigilant to uncertainty and took corrective action by enacting heightened levels of infection control. In other words, the healthcare team played a key role in thwarting the SARS threat in Vancouver, BC. Their system of accountability had implicitly embedded key complexity principles of interconnected systems, emergence, relationship-rich networks, shared sensemaking, and collaborative and facilitative leadership, thus enabling the system to effectively deal with uncertainty. They influenced the economic and workload gradients in a way that kept the operating point in a safe place.

Conclusion

This paper began with the idea that true accountability is impeded when nurse managers treat paradoxes of accountability within traditional evaluation frameworks. The paradoxes we highlighted were: 1) efficiency and effectiveness, 2) task and relationship, and 3) stability and change. We acknowledge the usefulness of traditional accountability frameworks, such as the balanced score card, to address one side of these paradoxes: efficiency, task, and stability. We also believe that Complexity Science complements these traditional approaches by drawing attention to the other side of the paradoxes: effectiveness, relationships, and change, including emergence. We suggest that nurse managers take a different path to managing the paradoxes of accountability by using both the traditional and complexity-informed approaches to evaluation. Integration of complexity and traditional approaches will help nurse managers develop a more comprehensive understanding of their work environment and manage the paradoxes of accountability in ways that will keep the operating point safe.

Accountability for nurse managers is laden with paradox. Just like the Möbius band, apparent opposites co-exist. To be truly accountable at the highest and most appropriate level for healthcare, nurse managers need to accept paradox as normal and embrace approaches which allow them to be accountable for the full range of their responsibilities.

Deborah Tregunno, PhD, RN, is assistant professor in the School of Nursing, Faculty of Health, York University. Prior to joining the School of Nursing, she completed a Canadian Health Services Research Foundation Postdoctoral Fellowship in the Faculty of Nursing, University of Toronto where she examined the link between performance measurement and a culture of patient safety. Her research interests focus on the field of quality and patient safety in critical care and other healthcare settings. Dr. Tregunno works with researchers from multiple fields to study complex organizational questions and contributes to a more comprehensive understanding of the organizational determinants of patient safety outcomes.

Brenda Zimmerman, PhD, CA, MBA, BSc, is professor of strategic management at Schulich School of Business, York University, Toronto. She is the founder and director of the Health Industry Management Program for MBA students. Her volunteer commitments in healthcare include service on the Science Advisory Board of Plexus Institute, membership on an advisory committee of the Canadian Royal College of Physicians and Surgeons, service as an advisor to the Canadian Public Health Agency; and membership on the Board of Mount Sinai Hospital in Toronto. Her latest co-authored book, *Getting to Maybe: How the World is Changed* is a Canadian best seller. She is also co-author of *Edgeware: Insights from Complexity Science for Health Care Leaders.*

Works Cited

1. M. Emmer, "Visual Art and Mathematics: The Moebius Band," *Leonardo* 13, no. 2 (1980): 108-111, 110.

2. A. Picard, "'Mommy, Are You Going to Die?'," *The Globe and Mail National Newspaper*, 2003, 5 April edition, sec. A.

3. Canadian Tourism Commission, "The Impact of Spring 2003 Events on U.S. Pleasure Travel to Canada," 2008. Available from http://www.corporate.canada.travel/docs/research_and_statistics/industry_research/CTC_Iraq-SARS_Impact_Summary%20-%20Eng.pdf.

4. Institute of Medicine and Committee on Quality of Healthcare in America, *Crossing the Quality Chasm: A New Healthcare System for the 21st Century* (Washington D.C.: National Academies Press, 2001).

5. L. Aiken, H. Smith, and E. Lake, "Lower Medicare Mortality Among a Set of Hospitals Known for Good Nursing Care," *Medical Care* 32, no. 8 (1994): 771-787.

6. A. Torangeau et al., "Nursing-Related Determinants of 30-Day Mortality for Hospitalized Patients," *Canadian Journal of Nursing Research* 33, no. 4 (2002): 51-70.

7. R. Morjikian, B. Kimball, and J. Joynt, "Leading Change," *Journal of Nursing Administration* 37, no. 9 (2007): 399.

8. A. Minnick, K. Pischke-Winn, and M. B. Sterk, "Introducing a Two-Way Wireless Communication System," *Nursing Management* 25 (1994): 42-47.

9. M. K. Pabst, J. C. Scherubel, and A. F. Minnick, "The Impact of Computerized Documentation on Nurses' Use of Time," *Computers in Nursing* 14 (1996): 25-30.

10. L. O'Brien-Pallas et al., "Developing and Testing a Model to Predict Outcomes of Organizational Change," *Nursing Economics* 15 (1997): 171-182.

11. L. Aiken and P. Patrician, "Measuring Organizational Traits of Hospitals: The Revised Nursing Work Index," *Nursing Research* 49 (2000): 146-153.

12. E. T. Lake, "Development of the Practice Environment Scale for the Nursing Work Index," *Research in Nursing & Health* 25 (2002): 176-188.

13. B. Berney and J. Needleman, "Impact of Nursing Overtime on Nurse-Sensitive Patient Outcomes in New York Hospitals 1995-2000," *Policy, Politics and Nursing Practice* 7, no. 2 (2006): 87-100.

14. J. Spetz, "California's Minimum Nurse-to-Patient Ratios," *Journal of Nursing Administration* 34, no. 12 (2005): 571.

15. E. Kurtzman and J. Corrigan, "Measuring the Contribution of Nursing to Quality, Patient Safety and Healthcare Outcomes," *Policy, Politics and Nursing Practice* 8, no. 1 (2007): 20-36.

16. J. Needleman, E. Kurtzman, and K. Kizer, "Performance Measurement of Nursing Care," *Medical Care Research and Review* 64, no. 2 (2006): 10S-43S.

17. C. Piedalue F. Goode, "Evidence-Based Clinical Practice," *Journal of Nursing Administration* 9, no. 6 (1999): 15-21.

18. C. Stetler, *Evidence-Based Practice and the Use of Research: A Synopsis of Basic Concepts and Strategies to Improve Care* (Washington, D.C.: Nova Foundation, 2001).

19. B. Melnyk and E. Fineout-Overholt, *Evidence-Based Practice in Nursing & Healthcare* (Philadelphia: Lippincott Williams & Wilkins, 2004).

20. J. Plouffe and C. Seniuk, "Walking the Walk: Living Evidence-Based Practice," *Dynamics* 15, no. 1 (2004): 14-17.

21. A. Kitson, G. Harvey, and B. McCormack, "Approaches to Implementing Reasearch in Practice," *Quality in Healthcare* 7 (1998): 149-159.

22. L. Pierce, "Evidence Based Practice in Rehabilitation Nursing," *Rehabilitation Nursing* 32, no. 5 (2007): 203-210.

23. S. Seaman, "Interdisciplinary Approach to a Total Knee Replacement Program," *Nursing Clinics of North America* 35, no. 3 (2000): 405-415.

24. S. Winch, A. Henderson, and D. Creedy, "Read, Think, Do!: A Method for Fitting Research Evidence into Practice," *Journal of Advanced Nursing* 50, no. 1 (2005): 20-27.

25. C.A. Estabrooks et al., "Individual Determinants of Research Utilization: A Systematic Review," *Journal of Advanced Nursing* 43 (2003): 506-520.

26. H. Thompson, C. Kirkness, and P. Mitchell, "Fever Management Practices of Neuroscience Nurses, Part II: Nurse, Patient and Barriers," *Journal of Neuroscience Nursing* 39, no. 4 (2007): 196-205.

27. R. Newhouse et al., "Evidence-Based Practice: A Practical Approach to Implementation," *Journal of Nursing Administration* 35, no. 1 (2005): 35.

28. C. Burnes, "Development and Content Validity Testing of a Comprehensive Classification of Diagnoses for Pediatric Nurse Practitioners," *International Journal of Nursing Terminologies and Classifications* 2, no. 3 (1991): 93-104.

29. C. Orchard, C. Reid-Haughian, and R. Vanderlee, "Health Outcomes for Better Information and Care (HOBIC): Integrating Patient Outcome Information into Nursing Undergraduate Curricula," *Canadian Journal of Nursing Leadership* 9, no. 3 (2006): 28-33.

30. D. Tarlier, "Beyond Caring: The Moral and Ethical Bases of Responsive Nurse-Patient Relationships," *Nursing Philosophy* 5, no. 3 (2004): 230.

31. P. Benner and J. Weubel, *The Primacy of Caring* (Menlo Park: Addison-Wesley, 1989).

32. L. Ginsburg and D. Tregunno, "New Approaches to Interprofessional Education and Collaborative Practice: Lessons From the Organizational Change Literature," *Journal of Interprofessional Care* 19, no. Supplement 1 (2005): 177-187.

33. I. Ajzen and M. Fishbein, *Understanding the Attitudes and Predicting Social Behavior* (Englewood Cliffs: Prentice-Hall Inc., 1980).

34. D. E. Pathman et al., "The Awareness-to-Adherence Model of the Steps to Clinical Guideline Commpliance. The Case of Pediatric Vaccine Recommendations," *Medical Care* 34, no. 9 (1996): 873-890.

35. D. Gustafson et al., "Developing and Testing a Model to Predict Outcomes of Organizational Change," *Health Services and Research* 38 (2003): 751-776.

36. J. Olsson et al., "Developing and Testing a Model to Predict Outcomes of Organizational Change," *Quality Management in Healthcare* 12 (2003): 240-249.

37. B. Schneider and C. Goldwasser, "Be a Model Leader of Change," *Management Review* 87, no. 3 (1998): 41-45.

38. J. G. Paolillo and W. B. Brown, "How Organizational Factors Affect R&D Innovation," *Research Management* 21 (1978): 12-15.

39. D. M. Rousseau and A. Tijoriwalas, "What's a Good Reason to Change? Motivated Reasoning and Social Accounts in Promoting Organizational Change," *American Psychological Association* 84, no. 4 (1999): 514-528.

40. J. REason, "Achieving a Safe Culture: Theory and Practice," *Work and Stress* 12 (1998): 293-306.

41. L. R. Goldberg, "The Structure of Phenotypic Personality Traits," *American Psychologist* 48 (1993): 26-34.

42. M. Farjoun and B. Zimmerman, "What Hospitals Can Do to Fight the Next SARS-like Crisis," *The Globe and Mail National Newspaper*, 2007, sec. A.

43. Vancouver Coastal Health Research Institute, "Drs. Roscoe and Purssell and Ms. S. Scharf Accepted an Award of Excellence from the BC Centre for Disease Control and the Office of the Provincial Health Officer on behalf of VGH for Early Recognition and Response to Patient Zero of SARS," 2008. Available from http://www.vchri.ca/s/Triumphs_Honours_Awards2003.asp?ReportID=74550&_Title=Drs.-Roscoe-and-Purssell-and-Ms.-S.-Scharf-accepted-an-Award-of-Excellence-.

44. F. Westley, B. Zimmerman, and M. Quinn Patton, *Getting to Maybe: How the World is Changed* (Mississauga: Random House Canada, 2006), 9.

45. R. Kaplan and D. Norton, "The Balanced Scorecard: Measures That Drive Performance," *Harvard Business Review* 7, no. 1 (1992): 71-79.

46. J. Cutright, S. Stolp-Smith, and E. Edell, "Strategic Performance Management: Development of a Performance Measurement System at the Mayo Clinic," *Journal of Healthcare Management* 45, no. 1 (2000): 58-68.

47. L. Biro, M. Moreland, and D. Cowgill, "Achieving Excellence in Veterans Healthcare — A Balanced Scorecard Approach," *Journal of Healthcare Quality* 25, no. 3 (2003): 33-39.

48. Ontario Hospital Association and The Government of Ontario. Hospital Report 2001: Emergency Department Care. 2001. Toronto, Hospital Report Research Collaborative.

49. D. Gordon et al., "Hospital Management Decision Support: A Balanced Scorecard Approach," *Medinfo* (1998): 453-456.

50. L. McGillis Hall et al., "Nurse Staffing Decision Making Models: Canadian Perspecitves," *Policy, Politics and Nursing Practice* 11, no. 7 (2006): 261-269.

51. D. Tregunno et al., "Competing Values of Emergency Department Performance: Balancing Multiple Stakeholder Perspectives," *Health Services Research* 4, no. 39 Part 1 (2004): 771-791.

52. J. A. Gamble, *A Developmental Evaluation Primer* (The J.W. McConnell Foundation, 2007).

53. R. Cook and J. Rasmussen, "Getting Solid: A Model of System Dynamics and Consequences for Patient Safety," *Quality and Safety in Healthcare* 14 (2005): 130-134.

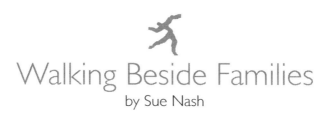

Walking Beside Families
by Sue Nash

The power of nursing is not in the ability to effect change, rather, by joining into the relational flow of health that families are living, the power to change emerges.[1]

Introduction

A journey through complexity naturally leads us into the land of families. Classic texts on family nursing present models of assessment grounded in a systems and reductionistic based approach—taking apart the structures and functions of a family to assess when and how nurses should intervene.[2-6] These models attempt to explain the construction of families, but do not shed enough light on the diverse relationships within the family or on outcomes that appear when people interact and co-evolve.

The purpose of this chapter is to explore family nursing in light of Complexity Science. Taking a historical perspective, I review the traditional groundings of family nursing, taking into consideration the contributions made by family social science, family therapy, and nursing theory. In light of new understandings grounded in Complexity Science, families are examined as examples of complex adaptive systems (CASs). I will explore families through a lens that recognizes families as emerging, creative, unpredictable, and ever-changing. The implications of a shift from the familiar traditional model of family assessment and intervention to a practice grounded in Complexity Science will be explored.

Family Nursing

Family nursing happens whenever the family is encountered, whether as a unit or as individual members. Traditionally, family nursing involved caring for the patient within the context of the family, or caring directly for the family as a whole, as is integral in pediatrics, obstetrics, and geriatrics.[4] Public health, psychiatric, and transcultural nursing have a rich tradition of the "family as client" model of care.[5;7-9] Family nursing offers an opportunity to promote health by encouraging family members to support one another.

Evolving Definition of Family

Family can be conceptualized in a variety of ways. *Nuclear family* originally referred to "a married man and woman with their offspring,"[10] and is now associated with what is often considered the traditional family, consisting of a mother, father, and children related by blood and living in a shared household.[11;12] The U.S. Census Bureau's[13] legal definition of family as a formal unit consisting of two or more persons related by birth, adoption, or marriage reflects these earlier notions of family. The U.S. Census Bureau recently expanded this definition to include those informally related by choice.[14]

By the late 1990s and early in the new millennium authors on family nursing theory began to recognize that the family is self-defined by its members, reflecting the trend of a more personal rather than societal definition of family.[3-6;14-16] According to these more modern theorists, this includes whomever the family considers significant, and membership may be based on marriage, partnership, blood lines, legal contracts, or emotional bonds. For example, families may include caring networks, extended multigenerational networks, blended families, or clans. Family members may be physically present or absent due to separation, divorce, schooling,

Table 1: Domains informing family nursing

	Family social science	**Family therapy**	**Nursing theories**
Purpose	To describe and explain family dynamics—focus on the literal family	To describe dysfunction and prescribe treatment	To guide nursing practice
Focus	Interdisciplinary approach focused on adaptation and change	Family therapy	Nursing care / patient care
Target	Normal families	Troubled families	Healthy and ill families focusing on health promotion

marriage, work commitments, war, immigration, estrangement, incarceration, or even death. However defined, families are part of an intricate web of emotional involvement and support.

Traditional Approaches to Family Nursing

Family nursing draws on knowledge from several disciplines, building on theory and research from family social science, family therapy, and nursing. Table 1 summarizes the major characteristics of each of these three disciplines.

Family Social Science

Family social science uses an interdisciplinary approach that draws on knowledge from family sociology, social work, psychology, and education in explaining how normal families work and interact. Family developmental theory is one branch of family social science which is grounded in systems theory. Family developmental theory defines family in terms of *structure, function,* and *developmental processes.*[4;5;17] Structure refers to the overall organization of the family and is associated with communication patterns, power structures, role structures, and values.[5;6;8] When nursing practice is based on this framework, nurses assess informal and formal family roles, role modeling and flexibility of role assignment, and role assumption. It is assumed that identifying "who does what" in a family helps the nurse know how to best individualize care. Family functions include affective functions (the family's response to member needs), socialization functions, and healthcare functions. Developmental stages are viewed as occurring in a predictable and sequential manner.[18-20] While family theorists now recognize that these stages are not rigid and each family is unique, the concept of family defined in terms of sequential stage development remains predominant in family nursing literature.[4;5;21] In recent years family literature has reflected a growing recognition that families are neither static in form nor clearly sequential in their developmental patterns.[20;22]

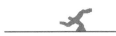

All nursing is family nursing and interaction between the nurse and the family is central to nursing practice.

With new insights into the interconnected nature of human beings, contemporary family theorists have moved from a developmental stage and task model to a perspective that takes into consideration the history and context that shape family growth and development.[23;24] This more holistic view, which is referred to in the literature as a "life course perspective," increasingly recognizes the dynamic nature of ongoing family interactions and relationships.[25] It also recognizes that the family is the classroom for cultural beliefs and norms, and reflects the culture's individualistic or collectivist belief system.[14;26-30]

Family Therapy

Family therapy builds on concepts and principles from family social science and psychology, offering major insights into family communication patterns. Family therapy has its roots in family systems theory, which was first developed by Murray Bowen.[31] Bowen considered the family to be an emotional system in which coping strategies and patterns are passed from one generation to the next in a process called multigenerational transmission. Family therapy also focuses on interactions and relationships among family members and how those relationships manifest as patterns within families. Contemporary family therapy theories advocate complex models that take into account socioeconomic, cultural, gender role, and religious experiences in addition to developmental stages. The shift from a view of the family as a rigid system with specific structures and developmental stages advocated by family social science to the focus on interaction, relationships, and patterns of communication seen in Bowen's family systems theory demonstrates a growing appreciation for the complex nature of family interactions.

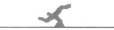

It is clear there is a gap between what family nursing education has taught about how families should behave and how families actually behave.

Nursing Theory

Because most nursing theories focus on the individual patient, their contribution to family nursing is mostly inferred. Martha Rogers was the first nursing theorist to discuss the significance of patterns of interaction between individuals.[32-34] Margaret Newman built on these insights and included family as part of the patterns of energy she considers the focal point for nursing care.[35;36] Newer nursing practice models, including Hartrick Doane and Varcoe's[37] model of family nursing as relational inquiry, continue to be developed. These more recent models emphasize the importance of relating and interacting with clients and families. As Hartrick Doane and Varcoe[37] point out, all nursing is family nursing and interaction between the nurse and the family is central to nursing practice.

Current family researchers advocate an interdisciplinary approach to the family that recognizes the complex patterns of interaction associated with families.[38;39] Control has shifted or perhaps returned to its rightful place. We are beginning to recognize that "the power of nursing is not in the ability to effect change, rather, by joining into the relational flow of health that families are living, the power to change emerges."[37]

As noted above, family nursing has traditionally viewed the family through a mechanistic lens which focused on family structure and family developmental stages. These theories instruct the nurse to take the family apart to see the whole.[14;40] There is a focus on helping the family by fixing the broken "parts." These approaches have met with limited success. It is clear there is a gap between what family nursing education has taught about how families should behave and how families actually behave. In addition, there is a discrepancy in how much control nurses think they have versus how much they actually have. Complexity Science provides new insights into how we can address these gaps. Using a Complexity Science lens, patterns of interaction begin to stand out in greater clarity, and implications for a new way of envisioning family nursing are revealed.

Complexity Science and Family Nursing

Families as Complex Adaptive Systems (CASs)

Families are examples of CASs. Applying Zimmerman, Lindberg, and Plsek's[41] definition of CASs, one can see the family as a diverse system of interconnected components able to alter, change, and learn. Rather than view the family as comprised of systems, functions, and structures, Stacey[42] presents families as patterns of relating and interacting. The family is a CAS that interacts and co-evolves in complex, interconnected processes. Viewed through a Complexity Science lens, one sees family as emerging, transforming, and self-organizing.[43;44]

Assumptions Informing Family Nursing

Five assumptions grounded in Complexity Science inform an understanding of families. *The first assumption is that all people are interrelated, and nothing exists outside of a relationship to others.* Traditional family nursing teaches us that people are interrelated and assumes that there are predictable elements to the interactions among them. New insights grounded in Complexity Science clarify and expand this understanding, teaching us that everything is relational and recognizing that any time human beings interact, there is unpredictability and the potential for emergence of new patterns. When a family expands, for example by adding a new child, new configurations occur. Roles change and the family adapts and new patterns of responding develop. Complexity Science-based family nursing practice helps the nurse understand that families are dynamic systems composed of interacting and interdependent elements. Complexity Science-based family nursing also recognizes that relationships are the essence of the family-nurse interaction. From a Complexity Science perspective, to be effective in providing care to families, nurses must enter into relationship with the family and its individual members.

This view of families as CASs is in stark contrast to the traditional view of family nursing. The traditional family nursing paradigm places nurses in a paradoxical situation of providing care for patients without caring too much. It teaches that becoming emotionally involved would interfere with our professional responsibility and might even lead to burnout.[37] This is one of the fundamental paradoxes in nursing. Family nursing from a Complexity Science perspective holds that when nurses are open to knowing and caring for their patients and families, the potential for a treasured relationship exists.

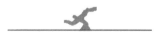

Reliance on reductionism has left us with a bunch of parts and no idea how to get them back together.

Relationships enrich the family-nurse interactions and bring meaning to nursing practice. The following story was shared with me by a seasoned nurse colleague and is an example of the tension between the tradition of professional detached care and Complexity Science-based relational nursing. The nurse had cared for a little boy and his father during a three-month period following a horrible automobile accident that claimed the life of the little boy's mother and two siblings. Six months after the child's discharge, the nurse was asked to attend the little boy's birthday party to celebrate the little one's life. He went. When his peers heard about it, he was chastised for not maintaining a professional distance. He stated, "For so long I was taught to hold back, not get overly emotionally involved. We'd been taught that getting too involved was unprofessional. Only when I allowed myself to truly care and truly feel the pain of the families I cared for did I experience the true meaning of what it means to be a nurse. …this is what I was called to do!" People are relational beings.[37] It is through interaction and caring that our practice takes on meaning.

The challenge for the nurse is to be able to be in relationship with the family while being able to reflect on the essence of the lived experience of the client. Norbert Elias[45] and Ralph Stacey[42] refer to being in relationship yet able to be outside of the relationship as involved detachment or detached involvement. This is another example of paradox at play—being able to be in relationship and simultaneously to be able to reflect on the nature of what it means to be in relationship.

The second assumption is that the sum of the parts is more than and different from the whole. Barabarsi[46] points out that reliance on reductionism has left us with a bunch of parts and no idea how to get them back together. Nurses were trained to study the roles, rules, functions, and structures of families, but the whole proved illusive. Rather than pulling a system apart to examine the pieces, it is "by comprehending the whole, the parts become meaningful."[47]

An example of the misunderstandings that can come from taking the "parts" out of context of the whole is seen in the following story. Teen moms in our society are often judged quite harshly. Nurses, as well as other individuals, are quick to indict teenaged moms as irresponsible, or even negligent, particularly when they judge the young woman without understanding the context of her decisions and her life. Expectations for teen moms and their infants in the U.S. include a life of poverty, abuse, and neglect.

One young family I cared for included a seventeen-year-old with a new baby who was participating in a school-based parenting program. On the surface, this young mother appeared to meet many of the negative stereotypes attributed to adolescent parents. She was young, poor, and had not finished her high school education before she became pregnant. Without consideration of the whole context of her life, it appeared that the future prospects for her and her infant were grim. However, looking at this teen in the context of her culture and her family provided a different picture. This adolescent was born into the Hmong culture. She was married at age 15, in a culturally sanctioned marriage arranged by her parents and her husband's parents. At the time of her marriage, her husband was 19, had finished high school, and was able to work full-time to support his family. Her pregnancy was not a result of a mistake or misjudgment but was planned. She was supported during her pregnancy and in caring for her infant by both her mother and her mother-in law. Family expectations were that she would complete her schooling with support from family caregivers. For this family, the birth of the baby to the young parents was considered timely and a reason to celebrate.

Viewing this teen through a Complexity Science lens, that is, widening our view to look beyond her age and poverty and allowing ourselves to see the whole context of her life, her abilities, her culture, and her support system, provides a very different picture from the one you would get in viewing her through a narrower lens. Seeking the whole picture rather than focusing on the individual "parts" of a patient's life story allows healthcare providers to better understand the strengths and abilities of each individual and family. This in turn allows nurses to better support families in moving forwards toward their health goals.

The third assumption grounded in Complexity Science is that change is nonlinear and disorderly. Cilliers[48] points out that change in systems is unpredictable, unexpected, and often surprising. Complex adaptive systems are unpredictable, co-evolving, and self-organizing.[41;44] Families demonstrate these same characteristics. As presented earlier in this chapter, family social science's traditional developmental stage theory has begun to be replaced by a life course perspective that recognizes that change is not predictable. Contemporary family theorists call for paying attention to the historical and cultural traditions influencing family style and redefining what is perceived as normal.[21;21;49]

Using Complexity Science as a means of conceptualizing family nursing allows us to direct our attention to the characteristics of complexity that lie within the system called family.[50;51] It offers insights into the nonlinear dynamics of relationships, building on the significance of initial conditions and the potential unpredictable effects of small changes, events, actions, and differences in perceptions and attitudes.[52] For example, a nurse might work for weeks with a family, putting in a large amount of effort to try to help them make needed changes with little success. At the same time, in working with another family, a very small act might lead to dramatic actions and positive life changes for them. Often nurses have been amazed at the seemingly small intervention that creates that "ah ha" reaction within the family. Instead of viewing families as systems that move through predictable stages and phases, it is important to recognize that movement and growth are nonlinear and disorderly. Real families do not fit into the models of family presented in traditional family theory, nor do they neatly follow the family developmental stages these theories propose. In reality, a family is often a messy unit consisting of a combination of individuals which may include parents, children, aunts, uncles, other relatives, and dear friends. Behavior of individuals within the family unit is unpredictable, and their actions can be surprising. The fact is that families do not act or react with the "same degree of predictability as machines."[53]

The fourth assumption is that new order emerges out of change. Boss[54;54] points out that families change throughout their lifespan. All families are dynamic, open, and interacting processes and it is through change that new structures emerge. Periods of order and disorder coexist, and therein lies the tension that is so uncomfortable for families and family nurses to face. Understanding this dynamic can be quite freeing for a family. For example, in my role as a parent educator, I counseled a single mother of four "tweens" and teens whose family life was constantly in a dramatic state of disorder. She stated that when she finally realized that these dramatic times were indicative that change was about to happen, she was able to let go and begin to trust the growth process that accompanied change. This insight allowed her to stop trying to prevent change and begin to allow her children the freedom to make choices and grow. It was through the disorder that new order emerged.

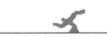

It is hard to be open to self-organizing patterns when one is using a fixed constellation or model for understanding a family.

Complexity Science helps nurses "develop a tolerance for ambiguity and uncertainty and 'hang in there' with clients until a new rhythm emerges."[55] Family nursing care built on this understanding will have relationships at its core and respect the family's dynamic processes of adapting, changing, and co-evolving.

Self-organization, emergence, and surprise are inherent in complex systems. It is hard to be open to self-organizing patterns when one is using a fixed constellation or model for understanding a family. In comparison to traditional approaches that use assessment tools to determine levels of family function, Complexity Science guides us to a focus on self-organizing processes and patterns. Looking at processes and emergent patterns through a Complexity Science lens reveals a huge array of family forms, strengths, and diverse family goals. Using the principles of Complexity Science, nurses can partner with families to build on their strengths, which are within and around the family. This co-evolving process means family and nurse are part of a mutual growth process. Box 1 describes a project a

Box 1: Conversation circles

There is a shift from "doing to" to accompaniment as new models of nursing emerge. One of these new nursing models has been implemented by Dr. Ruth Enestvedt, co-director of Augsburg College Nursing Center in Minneapolis, Minnesota. In order to change the conversation of healthcare by entering into collaborative partnerships with the homeless, safe spaces for conversation circles have been created at an inner city clinic for homeless individuals and families. Within the conversation circles, people who are homeless, nurses, politicians, and related healthcare workers begin to discover their collective strengths. This grassroots community building gives voice to the marginalized homeless people. Questions like: "What is needed to be healthy in the circumstances in which you live?" "What is working?" and "What do you need to make it work better?" lead people to share insights. Often in conversation, new ideas emerge. The next phase is to bring together representatives from service providers around the area to hear the stories of the people who live on the streets. There is a power shift and a focus shift. A partnership is created. The homeless people become the guides, expressing what they need, who they are, and describing their strengths and dreams. As the people who are homeless begin to discover new strengths, so too do the healthcare providers. In this manner, nurses and other healthcare provider come alongside and accompany the family on their journey in health (personal communication, April 9, 2008). ■

nursing school undertook that exemplifies the principle of nurses coming together with individuals and families to build strength, solve problems, and foster growth.

The fifth assumption is that history repeats itself-but not always. Family patterns and values tend to repeat themselves within and across generations. Families bring their history to the present and it shapes the future.[52] Families are situated in the everyday world in which they live and are constituted or shaped by the geo-political and social norms of their society.[37;48] Thus the legacy of the past shapes the future, but often in unexpected and surprising ways.[56] An example of a historical pattern that is perpetuated over generations is when victims of violence grow up to be perpetrators, such as when abused children grow up to be abusers.

Complexity Science also teaches that although every pattern has the potential to repeat itself, there is always potential for change. Although patterns are sustained by the behavior and actions of the agents, for the same reasons, these patterns can change. A seemingly small event can occur and shift everything, changing the patterns and creating a whole new meaning to a situation or event, or shift the family into a new way of being in relationship. The "casual" comment, "well, you know what happened to your grandfather don't you?" can reveal a history of depression and suicide that gives a whole new meaning to a generations' understanding of a parent's life course. This new insight offers the next generation options and choices for handling grief and sadness. Rowles writes of the reverberating consequences throughout the system as lives are "immersed in messy, complicated, interconnected systems that are not linear, static, or absolutely predictable."[57] Families share multigenerational patterns where members are influenced by each other, responding to changes of individuals within the family, sharing patterns, and being transformed. History matters but it does not necessarily control or predict. History can repeat itself, or new patterns and interactions can emerge, with different implications for the future.

Applying the principles of Complexity Science to families helps the nurse to more fully understand the dynamic nature of family. There is a shift in practice when we focus on relationships rather than problems. While the traditional approach to family nursing sees the dynamic, evolving, ever-changing nature of families as something that needs to be managed or controlled, nursing practice informed by Complexity Science brings new insights that give the nurse a fuller understanding of what is happening.

Complexity Inspired Family Nursing

What happens when nurses take Complexity Science seriously? How does nursing care change when practice is built on assumptions grounded in Complexity Science? Building nursing practice on the core principles of Complexity Science helps refocus care away from structure and function and toward relationships and interactions, and returns power to the family.

Recognize Diversity within Families

First, nurses should build on the diversity of family styles and resources. Traditionally, definitions of diversity focus on ethnicity. The first step is to expand the definition of diversity as related to families to include greater acknowledgement of who is and who is not a family member. For example, a family may be comprised of mother of two, and a grandmother. Another family may be comprised of a same-sex couple and their most supportive friends. A culturally-based social network or community may also be the family of care. Being open to what the family perceives itself to be allows the nurse to enter into relationship with family members on their own terms, building on the resources they bring and accepting their potential for growth and change. These concerns lead nurses to ask, "What is your relationship?" instead of asking, "Are you related?" It also leads nurses to refrain from supplying a plan of care developed in relative isolation and, instead, causes the nurse to work with the family by asking, "What would you like to gain out of this relationship?"

Break Away from Rigid Assessment Tools

The traditional patient interview format and assessment tools create boxes that frame our interaction with families. Nurses often come to the interaction with preconceived beliefs and go looking for what they expect to find. Simple words like *nuclear* and *extended* have embedded expectations of form and function. Complexity Science supports the fact that CASs self-organize and families create their own patterns, relationships, and ties. For example, a typical assignment in a family nursing course is to have the students create a genogram or family tree. In one of my family nursing courses, I gave my students this typical assignment. I explained the structure and the format and sent them on their way. One student's genogram challenged my understanding of family structure. Instead of the traditional tree-like structure made up of boxes, circles, lines, and arrows I expected, this student's diagram was a linear design filled with dotted lines to people in many directions. When I questioned her about it she smiled and said, "I'm from Sierra Leone, my family is a clan. These are my sisters and brothers." I learned something that day. The tools we use often boxed people into a specific world-view, denying them the right to express who they were. Using a complexity lens, I began to recognize self-organization as a process that is inherent in families.[44] Now I am asking students to draw their own picture of their family's patterns and interactions, without confining them to the assumptions and conventions embedded in a particular model.

Foster Diversity of Ideas, Strategies, and Connections

Rather than assuming that nurses have all the answers, Complexity Science teaches that by facilitating connections, families are strengthened and innovative options can come to be. One strategy open to family nursing is to build on the diversity of ideas within the family unit. A mother who participated in one of my parenting classes shared an example of the creative solutions that can arise when one is open to new ideas and approaches to solution finding. She reported that while visiting her local clinic one day, the nurse asked how things were going. This young mother expressed extreme frustration with her children and their continual bickering. The most recent concern was over a pair of cowboy boots. The six-year-old and four-year-old boys had decided that both of them wanted to own the boots. Every morning, the fight began. The mom was exhausted and this ongoing argument was the last straw. The nurse suggested they use a brainstorming session to enlist the kids in solution finding. She explained the process and the ground rules and sent the mom out, asking her to report back the next week. The mom called the nurse a few days later and reported, laughing, "You are not going to believe what those guys came up with! We had a 'meeting' and talked about it. We brainstormed, just like you told us to do. Now, each day one gets the right boot and the other gets the left boot! Can you believe it? We haven't had a fight in three days!" Over the next few months, the mom used this method in many other situations. She'd found a tool that was useful for dealing with her children's squabbles, and also re-discovered her sense of humor to see her through the rough days of raising four active children.

Diversity can also come in the form of resources and networking. Instead of relying only on the nurse as the expert, pulling in other voices can increase options and stimulate innovation. Family support groups are a wonderful forum for innovation to emerge. Box 2 describes how one such support group led to innovation and change in the way a family coped with their daughter's nighttime wandering. This story points out how important it is to help families establish new connections and relationships in times of stress.[44;46;58]

Box 2: Family support groups

In a group for families of special needs children that I led, the discussion turned to support and, frankly, exhaustion. The group was discussing social support and local networks. A young couple whose ten-year-old daughter had severe autism looked at each other and the wife began to quietly weep. Her husband reached out and grasped her hand. She said, "I can't leave my daughter with anyone. No one will take her. This is the only place we come to. This is our date night. My family has had it! They are no longer willing to help out. To make matters worse, we aren't getting sleep. She wanders the house all night. We take shifts and try to keep her locked in the room, but we discovered that she has learned to open the windows. What if she crawled out? What if she fell? Sometimes..." They grew quiet and the mother continued to weep.

One of the other mothers attending the group quietly asked if she'd explored a local fund that offers support for families with special needs children. She gave them the contact number and hints on how to fill out an application. The session ended and the parents agreed to talk on the phone during the next month. At our next meeting, this family shared that they were able to get some additional funding and it had changed their outlook. They had bought a large double bed built like a crib that would allow them to safely tuck their child in at night so they could get some sleep. They'd also applied for and received a grant for new windows that could be secured to keep their daughter inside the house. This networking didn't end here. This family became advocates at the local United Way, supported organization for parents with special needs, and began offering educational programs to teach others how to access funding. ∎

Box 3: Bringing down the silo walls

J.H. is a member of a local PTA leadership council in a town of about 100,000 people. In her community, the mental health of students has become a priority concern. To facilitate access to mental health services, the local PTA decided to host a series of seminars for parents and school employees highlighting local treatment resources for children suffering from depression. J.H. thought the best place to start was to gather information about existing services. She invited representatives from local service providers to discuss existing resources. Thirteen providers were contacted and all but one sent representatives. Each provider was asked to share information about services they provided and about perceived customer needs. J. H. shared with me that she was very nervous because she didn't know what to expect. Leaving it open to interaction and emergence was a risk, but it felt like the best way to hear what providers had to say.

Although the town thinks of itself as a small, close-knit community, much to the surprise of the organizers and participants, many of the providers had never met and none of the agencies had ever collaborated in such an endeavor. The other surprise was when J.H. shared the resources she had gathered, people began to notice errors. The brochures were outdated and the resources were thin. The challenge became how to get the correct information out to professionals and families. The silo walls began to fall. They talked and shared. They decided they would bring representatives from each of their agencies to the local school-based meetings and have time for roundtable discussions following the formal presentation. At the end of the meeting someone asked, "Next time can we talk about anxiety?"

Note: When J. H. shared this story with me I realized she had called together a complexity meeting. ■

Encourage Interaction among Diverse Professionals and Agencies

Often helping professionals and disciplines work in relative isolation from each other, even when working with the same families or client groups. This is sometimes referred to as "working in silos." It is important to the individuals and clients we work with to bring down the wall of these professional silos and to begin building interdisciplinary and inter-agency relationships. Box 3 includes a story of how people work in silos, isolated from each other, and the rewards of bringing those silos down. In this story, bringing people with diverse viewpoints together fostered new relationships and more inter-agency interactions. Richer insights were gained and new ideas emerged.

Pay Attention to Weak Links

Families with members who have weak links sometimes are more open to going outside their own frame of reference to discover new resources, to see their own strengths with a fresh perspective.

It is also important to remember the power of the weak link. Families are intricately networked with strong and weak links.[59-64] The strong links are those that have clearly defined roles, rules, and membership. Weak links are the casual or infrequent associations and relationships that individual and family members bring to the interaction.[59-61;61;63] An example of strong links include a closely-knit nuclear family. The weak links are friends and acquaintances that are known slightly but that have some influence. Complexity-inspired family nursing helps us understand that sometimes it is the weak link that makes the greatest contribution to the self-organizing process. While it seems counterintuitive, families that are not tightly bound by strong internal links often are more resilient and open to innovation from outsiders.[65] Families that have strong internal core links may be working within a narrow context and limited world-view. New ideas and ways of doing things brought into the family by individuals not closely tied to the family are examples of weak links that may change how families function. The Amish are an example of a self-referencing, strong internally linked group. They are often closed to outside resources and outside healthcare options.

"Weak ties play a crucial role in our ability to communicate with the outside world. To get new information, we have to activate our weak links."[46] Families with members who have weak links sometimes are more open to going outside their own frame of reference to discover new resources, to see their own strengths with a fresh perspective. They are open to outside referrals and outsider insights. The weak links principle guides

Box 4: The gift of presence: *three minutes of listening*

Students in Augsburg College's RN to BSN program often complain of having too little time to sit and listen to patient complaints or concerns. They have extremely demanding jobs and often feel overwhelmed by the ever-increasing amount of paperwork and documentation. The reality is that mandatory protocol and procedures often dictate how nurses should use their time. In an effort to promote relationships and refocus on the heart of nursing, students are challenged to enter into relationship with their clients by spending three minutes of focused presence—just listening and attending to the message being conveyed. They are told they will know who to interact with and are to report back the following class period. The experience is profound. One student shared the following story: The nurse was on morning rounds with the doctors. They entered the patient's room, asked the wife to step out, and drew the curtain around the bed to examine the patient. The doctors discussed the case and findings and periodically as they spoke the patient asked quietly if he could say something. The doctors were focused on the case and the need

to move along and just didn't hear him. As they exited the room, the patient tried a couple more times to get their attention, but they walked out. The student began to exit the room too, but remembered that she had class later that week and would have to share her three minutes of presence. She stopped and walked back into the patient's room. She stopped by his bed and said, "You said you wanted to say something. What was it you wished to ask?" The patient said, "Oh, I didn't want to ask anything, I just so wanted to thank them. They saved my life and I've been trying to thank them but they are always so busy!" The nurse and patient chatted for a few more minutes and then she walked around the curtain. There stood the wife with tears running down her face. She whispered the words "Thank you!" She said, "He has been so concerned. He just wanted them to know how grateful he is! Thank you." The student misted up as she shared this experience with the class. Three little minutes, so little time that meant so much.

the nurse to tune into the periphery of a family's network, looking for opportunities to bring in new perspectives and voices.

Nurses can create opportunities for interactions and connections. Nurses are network weavers, bringing people together. For example, they help families facing chronic illness to rally their support system and find ways to connect people to larger social networks. Nurses initiate care conferences, bringing all voices to the table. It is through increased opportunity to interact that linkages are created and emergence and innovation occur.

Remember that Change is Not Always Linear

Complexity Science advises that "small" can be very powerful. Researchers provide evidence that sometimes seemingly small actions or events can have profound impacts on systems.[66] Sometimes it is not about doing interventions to families, but rather it is about walking with the family on their journey through health and illness. Nurses who understand this principle realize that something as small as taking three minutes of time in their busy schedule to focus on and listen to their patient can profoundly impact their client's life. The client sees the nurse as engaged and caring and the nurse sees the client as a human being. Box 4 describes a brief interaction between an RN to BSN student and a patient and his wife. This story demonstrates how a brief interaction between the nurse and family members can make a profound difference

Another nurse shared how she spent some extra time one evening sitting by the bedside of her patient, letting him share his fears and concerns. Instead of reassuring him, she just sat and listened. She later shared, "Sometimes our patients can't see beyond the tragedy that faces them; they become their diagnosis and lose themselves in the process. When allowed to reminisce about life, they recognize their own purpose and reignite their will to survive." This nurse learned the lesson that it isn't always about having more time, but rather how we use the time we have. A few minutes of sharing the burden can be quite powerful. Box 5 tells the story of an RN to BSN student's interaction with an elderly widower and shows how profoundly a few minutes of interaction can affect both patient and nurse. The gift of time often seems like a small gift, but it can be a powerful building block in nurse-patient and nurse-family relationships.

Box 5: The power of listening

An RN to BSN student shared a classic example of the power of small actions. She wrote in an online posting, "I had a 23-hr observation patient who was 88 years old. He recently had a prostatectomy following prostate cancer and had a colonoscopy on the day of my shift. As I proceeded to introduce myself and do an assessment of him, I immediately found him to be a much younger acting and looking gentleman, more like a 60-year-old. I asked him if he had any family here with him from Iowa, and he thanked me for asking that question, stating that no one had asked him that today on this particular patient visit. As I was taking the adhesive tape off his wedding band, tears began running down his cheeks. He told me that his wife of 51 years, 7 months, and 20 days died a month ago and how much he missed her presence. He told of his deep respect for her as an accomplished pianist. He also told of his pact that he made with her that he would take care of his health so that he could finish her work before he would die. He also told of his regrets in not making a bigger effort to establish good relationships with his two grown children and not getting to know his grandchildren well.

As I listened to this man, I realized that he had lived a good and full life in some respects but still had regrets in other areas, areas that one cannot go back and do over. I felt a sense of sadness for him at this stage of his life to realize that his best friend was no longer at his side, and also could understand the emptiness that was present in his journey of life. As he was telling me about these events, I could see an immense amount of relief come over him and sensed a catharsis on his part. We visited for some time, and as I left my shift that night I really felt like I had connected with a patient in a significant manner" (E. Pochardt, personal communication, Sept. 20, 2007). ■

So What?

What does this mean to the practicing family nurse? How does nursing practice change when using a Complexity Science lens to inform practice? Begin by rethinking how nurses traditionally work with families, especially in terms of hierarchy and control. For too long healthcare providers thought they had control. In *Giving Voice to What We Know*, Margaret Pharris[67] points out that power is already situated within the family and the community. It only needs to be acted upon. By stepping back from approaches based on protocols and procedures and refocusing on the patient, the family, and their ways of knowing, nurses can better assist individuals and families to find meaning in the experiences of health and illness. Using Newman's framework, we distinguish between knowledge and power, recognizing that power already is in the hands of the family.[67] This means entering into relationship without predetermined expectations and prescribed assessment tools that attempt to control and predict the direction of interactions. This can be emancipating for both the family and the nurse.[37;64] Nursing students are taught that by following the protocol, they can remain in control of the situation. Accepting the fact that nurses are not in control can be frightening. Nurses wonder about the implications of letting the individual or family be in control. However, entering into relationship with the family is most likely to empower the family to effect positive changes.

The nurse-family relationship should be encouraged to develop by listening rather than by intervening. Complexity Science principles help us to bring the relationship into focus. As one RN-BSN student put it, "I thought I was doing good nursing when I used therapeutic communications to get the patient to cooperate. Now I realize that I was never in relationship and I was missing the point. A good nurse is IN relationship. It isn't a means to an end, it is the end!" (C. Evans, personal communications, May 4, 2006). According to Hartrick Doane and Varcoe, nurses need to "let go of the old dominant attractor patterns (the nurse is all knowing) and listen to the client."[37] The act of listening before asking questions changes how nurses practice. Letting go of the need to control the outcome and trusting the adaptive system unleashes creative potential and leads to new understandings of family needs and dynamics.

When nurses view families through the lens of Complexity Science, they become open to accepting that each family has different meanings of health. For example, dying at home peacefully, surrounded by family and loved ones, is viewed as healing and healthy by one family. Having terminal cancer and being able to get out of bed to attend a granddaughter's wedding may be defined as healthy by another family.

Finally, Complexity Science fosters an environment that encourages linkages, networking, connecting, and interconnectedness. Complexity Science suggests that nursing care of individuals and families is unpredictable and disorderly. As Newman writes, "The responsibility of the nurse is not to make people well, or to prevent their getting sick, but to assist people to recognize the power that is within them."[47] Helping individuals and families to recognize their power is grounded in the power of connecting, interacting, and interrelating.

Conclusion

Family nursing is historically grounded in family social science, family therapy, and nursing theory. This chapter began with the question: What does family nursing practice look like when the focus shifts from the familiar model of family assessment and intervention toward a practice grounded in Complexity Science? Looking at families through this new lens provides nursing with fresh insights about how families work and interact. Families are recognized to be evolving, emerging, and ever-changing. Both family and nurse gain from this shift. Letting go of perceived control and entering into relationship frees the nurse to come alongside families on their journey through healthcare. Complexity Science brings us to the heart of family nursing, embracing the diversity and creativity that lies within family nursing.

Sue Nash, EdD, MSN, RN, CFLE, is program coordinator of Augsburg College Department of Nursing, Rochester branch. Her primary practice has focused on facilitation of young families in a variety of community health settings. She has had thirty years of experience teaching both at the community and college level. Dr. Nash teaches family nursing at the graduate and undergraduate level and participates in clinical immersion experiences in Guatemala, Mexico, England, and the Pine Ridge Indian Reservation. Dr. Nash co-chairs the Nursing and Complexity Network of Plexus Institute. Network members are devoted to exploring the implications of Complexity Science for nursing.

Works Cited

1. G. Hartick Doane and C. Varcoe, *Family Nursing as Relational Inquiry: Developing Health-Promoting Practice* (Philadelphia: Lippincott, Williams & Wilkins, 2005), 20, 200-201, 52.

2. C. McHenry and S. Price, *Families & Change: Coping with Stressful Events and Transitions* 3 ed. (Thousand Oaks: Sage Publications, Inc., 2005).

3. S. Harmon Hanson, V. Gedly-Duff, and J. Rowe Kaakinen, *Family Health Care Nursing* 3 ed. (Philadelphia: F. A. Davis, 2005).

4. P. Bomar, *Promoting Health in Families: Applying Family Research and Theory to Nursing Practice* (Philadelphia: Saunders, 2004).

5. M. Friedman, F. Bowden, and E. Jones, *Family Nursing: Research, Theory and Practice* 3rd ed. (Upper Saddle River: Prentice Hall, 2003).

6. J. Wright and M. Leahey, *Nursing and Families: A Guide to Family Assessment and Intervention* 4th ed. (Philadelphia: F.A. Davis, 2005).

7. A. Whall, "The Family as the Unit of Caring: A Historical Review," *Journal of Advanced Nursing* 14 (1986): 211-216.

8. C. Smith and F. Maurer, *Community Health Nursing: Theory and Practice* 2 ed. (Philadelphia: W.B. Saunders Co., 2000).

9. M. Leininger, "Theory of Culture Care Diversity and Universality," in *Nursing Theories and Nursing Practice*, ed. M. Parker. (Philadelphia: F.A. Davis, 2001), 361-367.

10. G. Murdock, *Social Structure* (New York: Free Press, 1949).

11. P. Brandon and L. Bumpass, "Children's Living Arrangements, Co-Residence of Unmarried Fathers, and Welfare Receipt," *Journal of Family Issues* 22 (2001): 3-26.

12. D. Demo, W. Aquilino, and R. Fine, "Family Composition and Family Transitions," in *Sourcebook of Family Theory and Research*, ed. V. Bengston et al. (Philadelphia: Sage, 2005), 119-142.

13. U.S. Census Bureau, "Current Population Survey - Definitions and Explanations," Available from http://www.census.gove/popluations/www.cps/cpsdef.htm.

14. B. Ingoldsby, "Family Origin and Universality," in *Families in Global and Multicultural Perspective*, ed. B. Ingoldsby and S. Smith. 2nd ed. (Thousand Oaks: Sage, 2006), 67-78.

15. C. Smith, "Global Families," in *Families in Global and Multicultural Perspective*, ed. B. Ingoldsby and S. Smith. 2 ed. (Thousand Oaks: Sage, 2006), 3-24.

16. J. Gubruim and J. Holstein, *What Is a Family?* (Mountain View: Mayfield, 1990).

17. A. Hall and R. Fagan, "Definition of System," in *Structure and Behavior*, ed. W. Buckley. (Chicago: John Wiley & Sons, 1969), 81-92.

18. E. Duvall and B. Miller, *Marriage and Family Development* 6th ed. (New York: Harper & Row, 1985).

19. M. Arndt and B. Bigelow, "Hospital Administration in the Early 1990s: Visions for the Future and the Reality of Daily Practice," *Journal of Healthcare Management* 52, no. 1 (2007): 34-45.

20. B. Carter and M. Mc Goldrick, *The Changing Family Life Cycle: A Framework for Family Therapy* (New York: Gardner Press, 1989).

21. D. Klein and J. White, *Family Theories: An Introduction* (Thousand Oaks: Sage, 1996).

22. S. Slater, *The Lesbian Life Cycle* (New York: Free Press, 1995).

23. G. Elder, "Time, Human Agency, and Social Change: Perspectives on the Life Course," *Social Psychology Quarterly* 57 (1994): 4-15.

24. R. MacMillan and R. Copher, "Families in the Life Course: Interdependency of Roles, Role Configurations, and Pathways," *Journal of Marriage and Family* 67 (2005): 858-879.

25. R. Bucx et al., "Intergenerational Contact and the Life Course Status of Young Adult Children," *Journal of Marriage and Family* 70 (2008): 144-156.

26. M. McGoldrick, "Ehtnicity, Culture Diversity and Normality," in *Normal Family Processes*, ed. F. Walsh. 2nd ed. (New York: Guildford Press, 1993), 331-336.

27. J. Meyer-Walls, K. Myers-Bowman, and G. Posada, "Parenting Practice Worldwide," in *Families in Global and Cultural Perspective*, ed. B. Ingoldsby and S. Smith. (Thousand Oaks: Sage, 2006), 147-167.

28. C. Coll, J. Surrey, and K. Weingarten, *Mothering Against the Odds: Diverse Voices of Contemporary Mothers* (New York: Guildford Press, 1998).

29. J. DeLoache and A. Gottlieb, *A World of Babies: Imagined Childcare Guides for Seven Societies* (New York: Cambridge University Press, 2000).

30. L. Samovar, R. Poter, and E. McDaniels, *Intercultural Communication* 11th ed. (Belmont: Thomson Wadsworth, 2006).

31. M. Bowen, *Family Therapy in Clinical Practice* (New York: Jason Aronson, 1978).

32. C. H. Ellenbecker, J. Fawcett, and G. Glazer, "A Nursing PhD Specialty in Health Policy: University of Massachusetts Boston," *Policy, Politics and Nursing Practice* 6 (2005): 229-235.

33. J. Fawcett, *Analysis and Evaluation of Conceptual Models of Nursing* 4th ed. (Philadelphia: F.A. Davis, 2000).

34. J. Fawcett, "Spouses' Experiences During Pregnancy and the Postpartum: A Program of Research and Theory Development," *Journal of Nursing Scholarship* 21, no. 3 (1989): 149-152.

35. C. Picard and D. Jones, *Giving Voice to What We Know: Margaret Newman's Theory of Health as Expanding Consciousness in Nursing Practice, Research, and Education* (Boston: Jones and Bartlett, 2005).

36. M. Newman, *Health as Expanding Consciousness* 2nd ed. (Mississauga: Jones and Bartlett, 1994), XV.

37. G. Hartick Doane and C. Varcoe, *Family Nursing as Relational Inquiry: Developing Health-Promoting Practice* (Philadelphia: Lippincott, Williams & Wilkins, 2005), 52.

38. J. Seltzer et al., "Explaining Family Change and Variation: Challenges for Family Demographers," *Journal of Family* 67, no. 4 (2005): 908-925.

39. N. A. Wetzel and H. Winawer, "School-Based Community Family Therapy for Adolescents at Risk," in *Comprehensive Handbook of Psychotherapy*, ed. F. W. Kaslow, R. F. Massey, and S. D. Massey. (Philadelphia: John Wiley & Sons, 2002), 205-230.

40. G. Becker, "A Theory of the Allocation of Time," *Economic Journal* 75 (1965): 493-517.

41. B. Zimmerman, C. Lindberg, and P. Plsek, *Edgeware: Insights from Complexity Science for Health Care Leaders* (Irving: VHA Inc., 2001).

42. R. Stacey, *Complexity and Creativity in Organizations* (San Francisco: Berrett-Kohler Publishers, 1996).

43. T. Smith and G. Stevens, "Emergence, Self-Organization, and Social-Interaction: Arousal-Dependent Structure in Social Systems," *Sociological Theory* 14, no. 2 (1996): 131-153.

44. A. Suchman, "A New Theoretical Foundation for Relationship-Centered Care: Complex Responsive Processes of Relating," *Journal of General Internal Medicine* 21 (2006): 40-44.

45. N. Elias, *The Society of Individuals* (New York: Continuum, 2001).

46. A. L. Barabasi, *Linked: The New Science of Networks* (Cambridge: Perseus, 2002), 43.

47. M. A. Newman, "Theory for Nursing Practice," *Nursing Science Quarterly* 7 (1994): 153-157.

48. P. Cilliers, *Complexity and Postmodernism: Understanding Complex Systems* (London: Routledge, 1998), 1.

49. V. Bengston and K. Allen, "The Life Course Perspective Applied to Family Over Time," in *Sourcebook of Family Theory and Methods: A Contextual Approach*, ed. P. Boss et al. (New York: Plenum, 1993), 469-499.

50. H. Simon, *The Sciences of the Artificial* 3rd ed. (Cambridge: The MIT Press, 1999).

51. G. Gioretti and B. Visser, "A Cognitive Interpretation of Organizational Complexity," *Emergence: Complexity and Organization* 6, no. 1-2 (2004): 11-23.

52. F. Reitsma, "A Response to Simplifying Complexity," *Geoforum* 34 (2003): 13-16.

53. D. Munday, S. Johnson, and F. Griffiths, "Complexity Theory and Palliative Care," *Palliative Medicine* 17, no. 4 (2003): 308-309, 303.

54. P. Boss, *Family Stress Management: A Contextual Approach* 2nd ed. (Thousand Oaks: Sage, 2002).

55. M. Newman, "The Rhythm of Relating in a Paradigm of Wholeness," *The Journal of Nursing Scholarship* 31, no. 3 (1999): 227-230.

56. M. Hoopes, "Multigenerational Systems: Basic Assumptions," *Journal of Family Therapy* 15 (1987): 195-205.

57. G. Rowles, "Habituation and Being in Place," *Occupational Therapy Journal of Research, Supplement* 20 (2000): 52S-67S, 61S.

58. K. Smith and D. Berg, *Paradoxes of Group Life: Understanding Conflict, Paralysis and Movement in Group Dynamics* (San Francisco: Jossey-Bass, 1987).

59. R. A. Anderson et al., "The Power of Relationship for High-Quality Long-Term Care," *Journal of Nursing Care Quality* 20, no. 2 (2005): 103-106.

60. H. Coleman, "What Enables Self-Organizing Behavior in Business," *Emergence: Complexity and Organization* 1, no. 1 (1999): 33-38.

61. N. Luhmann, *Observations on Modernity* (Stanford: Stanford Press, 1995).

62. N. Luhmann, *Social Systems* (Stanford: Stanford Press, 1990).

63. W. Medd, "Complexity in the Social World," *International Journal of Social Research Methodology* 5, no. 1 (2002): 71-81.

64. G. Morgan, *Images of Organization* (Thousand Oaks: Sage, 1997), 16.

65. M. Gravnovette, "The Strength of Weak Ties," *American Journal of Sociology* 78 (1973): 1360-1380.

66. E. Lorenz, *The Essence of Chaos* (London: UCL Press, 1995).

67. M. Pharris, "Engaging with Communities in a Pattern Recognition Process," in *Giving Voice to What We Know: Margaret Newman's Theory of Health As Expanding Consciousness in Nursing Practice, Research, and Education*, ed. C. Picard and D. Jones. (Boston: Jones and Bartlett, 2005), 83-94.

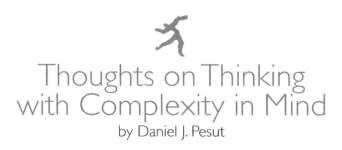

Thoughts on Thinking with Complexity in Mind
by Daniel J. Pesut

There is nothing as practical as a good theory.[1]

Introduction

Edward Tufte[2] in his book, *Beautiful Evidence*, observes the common analytic task in nearly all disciplines is to help people understand causality, make multivariate comparisons, examine relevant evidence, and assess the credibility of evidence and conclusions. There is an art, science, and complexity to the thinking that supports clinical reasoning. The purpose of this chapter is to introduce the Outcome-Present-State-Test (OPT) Model of Reflective Clinical Reasoning. The OPT model is a meta-model of clinical reasoning that has value for teaching clinical reasoning in nursing. The roles of critical, creative, and systems thinking and complexity principles in the reasoning process are described. The contribution of Complexity Science to the analysis and synthesis of systemic relationships of nursing care needs in a particular patient scenario is discussed. Conversations about the art, science, and complexities of clinical reasoning are likely to stimulate learning and promote effective clinical reasoning skills among faculty, students, and clinicians.

Framing Phenomena through Knowledge Representation

Clinical reasoning requires an understanding of the issue of knowledge representation in specific disciplines. Nearly every discipline uses knowledge representations or classification schemes that organize complex phenomena into understandable categories. Knowledge classification schemes provide discipline-specific clinical vocabularies. These clinical vocabularies become the content of clinical reasoning efforts. "Framing" a situation involves giving a meaning to a set of facts. Frames are mental models that help clinicians make sense of experience given a particular set of values, beliefs, theories, conceptual orientations, or discipline-specific worldviews.[3] Disciplines frame situations in different ways. Physicians frame issues in terms of disease and pathophysiology. Nurses frame issues in terms of people's responses to health states and conditions. Physical therapists frame issues in terms of function and rehabilitation. Social workers frame issues in terms of resources that help people manage social systems in which they live and work. Each of these frames is built on the professional identities, values, beliefs, theories, and conceptual frameworks of those individuals who operate within their disciplinary perspective. Reflecting on issues of framing in nursing and interdisciplinary work helps clarify disciplinary contributions and aids in achieving patient care goals and outcomes.

A number of clinical vocabularies are shared among disciplines. For example, many clinicians reason from a disease management frame of reference. Nurses may use the knowledge classification of nursing diagnoses (NANDA), interventions (NIC) and outcomes (NOC). Some nurses may choose to use the Seven Axis Model of the International Classification of Nursing Practice (ICNP). The World Health Organization (WHO) International Classification of Disease or the WHO International Classification of Functioning, Disability, and Health may be preferred by some. Many of these classification schemes are cross referenced in the Systematized Nomenclature of Medicine-Clinical Terms (SNOMED-CT). Classification schemes provide a conceptual, clinical, or disciplinary lens to view phenomena and help structure clinical thinking and reasoning. It could be argued that some differences of opinion arising in interdisciplinary teams are differences in knowledge representation and framing related to each discipline's phenomena of concern. One way to support interdisciplinary communication is to begin a dialogue about discipline-specific differences in knowledge representation or framing, and how differences in framing are complementary rather than competitive in patient care. As Davis, Shrobe, and Szolovits[4] note, "a theory of knowledge representation is a theory of reasoning." They write that knowledge representation "is a medium for pragmatically efficient computation, i.e., the computational environment in which thinking is accomplished." It helps us organize information appropriate inferences. It is, they write, "a medium of human expression, i.e., a language in which we say things about the world."[4]

Knowledge representation and the framing of nursing phenomena are complex and have evolved over time. The evolution of the nursing diagnosis movement best represents the nursing profession's commitment to knowledge representation of nursing problems, outcomes, and interventions. Concurrently with nursing knowledge representation and framing efforts, the manner in which clinical thinking and reasoning have been taught in nursing has evolved through time.

A Brief History of Clinical Thinking and Reasoning in Nursing

Prior to the 1950s, education in nursing was steeped in an apprenticeship model and care was based mainly on ritual, tradition, and standard operating procedures.[5] In the decades since the 1950s, the structure for clinical thinking has been based on the nursing process. Traditional nursing process, characterized by clinical thinking grounded in a problem solving model of assessment, planning, intervention, and evaluation (APIE), was designed to organize thinking to anticipate and quickly solve problems patients encountered. This first generation nursing process (1950–1970) structured clinical thinking through the frame of problem solving and emphasized the importance of assessment. Bio-psycho-social and physical assessments revealed deviations from accepted norms and thus triggered problem identification which was remedied by nursing actions, procedures, and interventions.

As problem solution patterns emerged, a small group of nurses began to recognize repetitive patterns of nursing concerns and problems. This attention to the pattern formation and relationships among nursing care needs in specific client populations stimulated a group of nurses to develop knowledge representation about issues of concern to nurses. These nurses appreciated the complexity of patient care needs and nursing remedies, and started to pay attention to patterns and relationships among behavioral cues, signs, and symptoms in addition to defining characteristics associated with patient responses to their own health and illnesses. This

Nursing diagnoses are knowledge representations that, define, explain, and describe patterns of behavior and patient responses to illness.

work evolved and nurses began to systematically represent, frame, and codify nursing phenomena into classification systems that have come to be known as nursing diagnoses, nursing interventions, and nursing outcomes. Nursing diagnoses are knowledge representations that, define, explain, and describe patterns of behavior and patient responses to illness. Pattern recognition and identification of relationships among cues, signs, and symptoms, and etiologies of these

indicators evolved into a classification system of nursing diagnoses referred to as NANDA (North American Nursing Diagnosis Association).[6] Meanwhile, work was also progressing on the systematic development of classification systems for nursing interventions known as the Nursing Interventions Classification (NIC) and nursing knowledge representations, related to framing of nursing sensitive outcomes known as the Nursing Outcomes Classification (NOC). Through systematic research, nurses created representations of nursing knowledge that frame the phenomena of concern for nurses.[7] Such work proved to be important for the development of nursing theory and practice.[8] Further information on the nursing classification taxonomies NIC and NOC can be found at the website of the Center for Nursing Classification & Clinical Effectiveness at the University of Iowa. This center can be found on the Internet at:

http://www.nursing.uiowa.edu/excellence/nursing_knowledge/clinical_effectiveness/index.htm.

There are important reasons to consider how the nursing knowledge representation work supports nursing scholarship.[9] These concurrent knowledge development processes help to frame clinical thinking and clinical reasoning in new ways. The development of nursing informatics and the move toward use of electronic health records makes continued attention to classification of nursing diagnoses, actions, and outcomes imperative because these classification systems help make nursing's impact on patient welfare visible. Such developments are likely to continue to have a great impact on nursing knowledge work in the twenty-first century.[10]

Attention to Diagnoses

As the issue of nursing diagnosis moved to the foreground, the four-step problem solving nursing process—assessment, plan, implement, evaluate (APIE)—changed. The knowledge representation and framing work related to nursing diagnoses created interest in the thinking that supports diagnostic reasoning. The four-step APIE model evolved into a five-step model with the acronym ADPIE – assess, diagnose, plan, intervene, and evaluate. By 1980, the ANA Social Policy Statement Nursing defined nursing as "the diagnosis and treatment of human responses to actual or potential health problems."[11]

The thinking strategies that enable one to perform clinical reasoning are gained through practice, conscious reflection, and attention to issues of complexity associated with a client's story and the context of practice.

In the mid 1990s, healthcare rules changed and the notion of outcome specification replaced problem identification. In fact, reimbursement rules were predicated on outcomes achieved, not necessarily problems identified. At the same time, interest in how novice nurses became expert nurses[12;13;14] became a popular topic of nursing research. These two movements led scholars to explore how nurses were thinking about their practice and how caring, reasoning, and moral imperatives influenced the development of expertise and clinical wisdom. "Knowing the patient" and blending scientific knowing with the unique characteristics and context of a patient's story enabled nurses to practice the science ~ art of nursing. The tilde (~) has been proposed as the new symbol to represent complementary pairs.[15]

Assessment and understanding of the client in context emerged as a priority. Interest in the nature and nurture of clinical reasoning and clinical thinking became a focus for nursing education, research, and practice.

Making the critical thinking in clinical reasoning explicit became an important topic, and criteria for assessing students and accrediting nursing education programs resulted.[16-19]

Clinical reasoning is supported by many types of thinking skills and strategies. The thinking strategies that enable one to perform clinical reasoning are gained through practice, conscious reflection, and attention to issues of complexity associated with a client's story and the context of practice. For a discussion on the importance of reflective practice in nursing, readers are directed to the Honor Society of Nursing, Sigma Theta Tau International as well as Burns and Bulman,[20] and Johns.[21] What follows is brief discussion about the Outcome-Present-State Test (OPT) Model of Reflective Clinical Reasoning and the critical, creative, systems, and complexity thinking that is involved in clinical reasoning.

The OPT model is a concurrent information processing model that is iterative, recursive, and nonlinear.

From Diagnoses to Outcomes

Outcome specification, although implied in the first two generations of nursing process, did not receive explicit attention in the ADPIE model. Work in outcome specification added to the nursing knowledge classification systems that organized nursing knowledge and made explicit the value and contributions of professional nurses to care and service.[22] Outcome specification was assuming increased importance in nursing education programs, leading Pesut and Herman[23] to create the Outcome-Present-State Test (OPT) Model of Reflective Clinical Reasoning. This model is based on their clinical teaching experiences with traditional and experienced RN to BSN students. The model puts emphasis on outcome specification given a presenting problem state and advocates the juxtaposition of a problem state and a specified desired state.

It seemed to Pesut and Herman[24] there was a need to create a model of clinical reasoning that embraced the complexity of the patient's story with attention to the complementary nature of the patient's identified problem and specified outcomes that could frame nursing care using existing knowledge representation and classification schemes. The complementary nature[15] of problems ~ outcomes provides nurses with clinical reasoning and nursing care insights. Examples of complementary pairs include: Pain ~ comfort, anxiety ~ anxiety control, suicidal ideation ~ will to live, self-care deficit ~ self care. The complementary nature of problem ~ outcomes reflects that nurses help people transition from states of illness to states of health.

The OPT model is a concurrent information processing model that is iterative, recursive, and nonlinear. This contrasts contemporary nursing process models which are often presented as information processing models that are linear and sequential. For example, the most recent description of nursing process offered by the American Nurses Association (ANA) describes a six-step process with four additional sub-sets of steps under the implementation phase of the nursing process: assessment, diagno-

In the moment to moment vigilance that nurses apply as they work and interact with patients, they are always updating the matrix of their thinking and reasoning about what is happening and how patients are responding.

sis, outcome specification, planning, implementation (including coordination of care, health teaching and promotion, consultation, prescriptive authority, and treatment), and evaluation.[25] However, such models cannot adequately represent the complex nature of nurses' clinical reasoning which is not simple but rather complicated or complex (see Lindberg and Lindberg chapter for explanation of this framework). Many patients' conditions change from hour to hour and sometimes from minute to minute. In the moment to moment vigilance that nurses apply as they work and interact with patients, they are always updating the matrix of their thinking and reasoning about what is happening and how patients are responding. As they plan and provide care, nurses constantly reason about patient conditions and nursing care needs. The Outcome-Present-State Test (OPT) Model of Reflective Clinical Reasoning provides structure, content, process, and strategies that help students and clinicians master the complexity of clinical reasoning.

Outcome-Present-State Test Model of Reflective Clinical Reasoning

The OPT model is a third generation (2000-2020) nursing process model that provides a structure for clinical reasoning that focuses on outcomes derived from considering the relationships among nursing care problems associated with a specific client story.[23] In this model, as relationships among nursing diagnoses are analyzed, patterns and meaning in the data and information help focus and define key aspects of patient nursing care needs. Building on the dynamic relationships among these competing nursing care needs leads to the identification of one or more keystone issues that are translated into a desired outcomes. Outcome specification supports the development of clinical judgment skills.

Complexity theory helps explain how many of the thinking and reasoning strategies that support the model can be understood and learned. What follows is brief discussion about the clinical reasoning that is supported by the model structure[23;24] and Pesut.[26;27] The OPT model provides

Figure 1: The OPT Model of Clinical Reasoning[23;24]

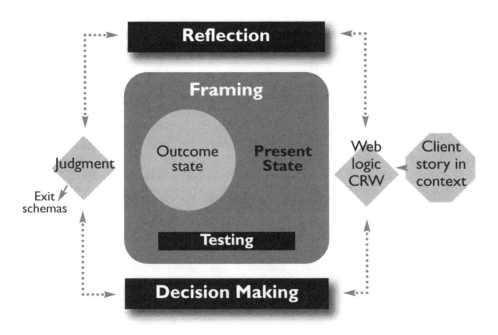

a structure for clinical thinking and reasoning. This model is illustrated in Figure 1. The main ingredients of the model are listed in Box 1.

Clinical reasoning involves concurrent, creative, critical, and systems thinking. Clinical reasoning is supported by both cognitive and metacognitive thinking skills.[28] Pesut and Herman created the OPT model and defined several thinking strategies that support the model. These include knowledge work, self-talk, framing, schema search, hypothesizing, if-then thinking, juxtaposition of present states with desired outcome states, testing, reflexive comparison, judgment, reframing, and reflection checks. The thinking strategies that enable one to perform clinical reasoning are gained

Box 1: Main elements of the OPT model

- Attention to the client story

- Discerning the role of framing in the client situation

- Mapping relationships among care needs in a clinical reasoning web (CRW).

- Identification and explanation of patterns of relationships among competing nursing care needs

- Simultaneous considerations include attention and reflection on multiple nursing diagnoses and their relationships with one another given the patients evolving story

- Iterative and recursive thinking about relationships between needs and attention to what emerges from this reflection

- Defining a present state and its complementary outcome state

- Determining a well-formed outcome

- Deciding on nursing interventions and clinical indicators of outcome achievement

- Making clinical judgments through iterative reflections on outcome achievement based on patient progress toward outcome criteria and clinical indicators that have been established through practice, conscious reflection, and attention to the client's story and its context.

The model advocates that clinicians *simultaneously* consider and understand relationships among competing diagnoses and consider the balancing and reinforcing loops and causal connections among the diagnoses. The OPT model provides structure, process, and strategies for considering patient stories in light of discipline-specific knowledge representations. Relating elements of the story in systematic ways requires application of critical, creative, systems, and complexity thinking. Complexity thinking is defined in this model as thinking derived from complexity principles and practices. These thinking strategies lead to framing, understanding of system dynamics, and ultimately the juxtaposition of present states with desired outcome states. Decision making leads to consideration of interventions that facilitate the transition from the defined present state to the desired outcome state. Judgments of outcome achievements are also a part of the OPT model.

Through stories, one can extract and communicate subtle aspects of expertise and develop pattern recognition.

Relationships among diagnoses are represented in a visual way with a tool called a Clinical Reasoning Web (CRW). Figure 2 is an example of a CRW. As patterns and relationships are identified and described, what often emerges is insight about the relationships among competing patient care needs. Iterative reflection and expressed relationships among multiple nursing care needs lead to the identification of one or more "keystone" issues that act as a leverage points in the system dynamic. A keystone issue is defined as a central supporting element of the client's story—derived from an analysis of system dynamics and the complexity of relationships among identified diagnoses. Once "keystone issue(s)" are determined, efforts are put into specifying the problem ~ outcomes associated with the complementary pair of issues that the "keystone problems ~ desired outcomes" represent. Evidence for outcome achievement is developed. Interventions are chosen and applied to help the client transition from the problem or presenting states to the desired or specified states.

Clinical decision making in this model is defined as choosing nursing actions. A clinical judgment is the conclusion or meaning one gives data drawn from a comparison of client present state data to specified outcome criteria. Reflection on judgments may suggest the need for reframing situations or creating new tests, making different intervention decisions or choices. Concurrently, the nurse engages in reflection and judgment about outcome achievement.

There are five iterative thinking sequences. There is the logic of the nursing diagnosis; the logic of relationships among competing diagnoses ~ outcomes; the logic of interventions that transitions client from present to desired states; the logic of patterns and relationships among problems, outcomes, and interventions; and finally, the logic of managing and self-regulating one's own thinking and reasoning efforts. A reasoning task, however, begins with understanding the patient's story.

Clinical Reasoning: The Patient Story

Initiation of reasoning tasks with the OPT model begins with a patient's presenting story. Why the story? Gary Klein[29] suggests stories are sources of learning because they help organize events into meaningful frameworks. He further notes that stories are natural experiments and help describe and link networks of causes to effects. Stories are like mental simulations. Through stories, one can extract and communicate subtle aspects of expertise and develop pattern recognition. Stories provide the big picture and help sensitize one to situation awareness and help pinpoint where one can use leverage points to solve poorly defined problems. Stories help people to develop judgment about a class of typical goals, courses of action, or the solvability of a problem. Stories also help people to make discriminations, detect gaps in plans of action, and detect barriers to plans and proposed solutions. Through consideration and inter-relating of the facts, clinicians discover patterns among competing patient care problems and needs. Thus, OPT is an iterative, recursive concurrent information processing model that requires clinicians to consider the cause and effect— balancing and reinforcing loops among numerous problems simultaneously. How might we go about illustrating this? The answer rests with the creation of a clinical reasoning web that helps to make the invisible dynamics among competing nursing care needs visible.

Representation of Complexity and Relationships through a Clinical Reasoning Web

To create a clinical reasoning web, one uses information gained from the patient's story. The condition the patient is coping with is put in the middle of the web and all the nursing care consequences (diagnoses) associated with that condition are represented as spokes of the web. The CRW visually represents the "web" of causal loop diagrams and helps explicate balancing and reinforcing connections among the diagnoses. Using the web as a reasoning tool, one begins to reflect and explain how each of the issues relates to or influences each of the other issues. Analysis of complex associations, balancing-reinforcing loops, and cause and effect relationships lead to the identification of one or more keystone issues in the complex system of patient care problems.

Use of a CRW promotes reflection on the patient's story as a whole rather than sequentially. Such thinking helps support understanding of the complexities involved in competing nursing care needs. This percolation leads to a phase shift or seeing the system dynamic in a new way. Albert

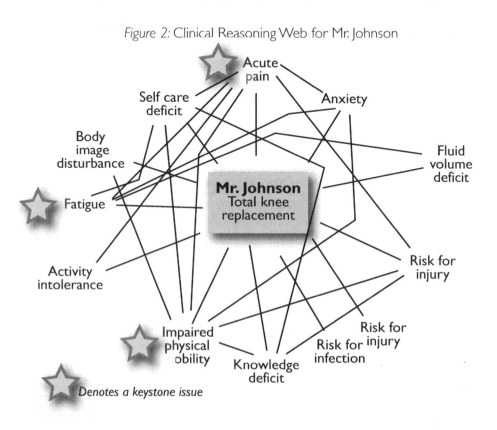

Figure 2: Clinical Reasoning Web for Mr. Johnson

Barabasi[30] suggests when we randomly pick and connect pairs of nodes together in a network, something special happens. Fitting the pieces to one another, node by node and link by link, capturing their dynamic interplay, results in a phase shift and a new pattern of linked relationships emerges. Combining systems thinking with an understanding of the complexity of relationships embedded in a particular patient story gives rise to the challenge of complexity thinking about how the patient as a system of care needs interacts and is affected by relationships with care providers and the context in which they live and work.

An Example - The Story of Mr. Johnson

Consider the story of Mr. Johnson who has just experienced bilateral knee replacements. Consider the nursing care consequences or the human responses Mr. Johnson is likely to experience as a result of his knee replacement surgery. Some of the actual or potential nursing diagnoses or issues include: pain, anxiety, risk for infection, fluid volume deficit, knowledge deficit, impaired physical mobility, and activity intolerance. In addition, he may also deal with fatigue, body image disturbance, and self-care deficit. The challenge is how one reasons about all of these issues concurrently. How does one begin to develop propositional knowledge about the multiple nursing diagnoses and how they interact, affect, and influence one an-

Table 1: Contrasting problems with outcomes for Mr. Johnson

Outcomes	Problems
• Comfort (pain control)	• Acute pain
• Anxiety control	• Anxiety
• Joint movement	• Impaired physical mobility
• Self-care	• Self-care deficit
• Ambulation	• Activity intolerance
• Endurance	• Fatigue
• Energy management	• Risk: infection, injury
• Risk control	• Knowledge deficit
• Knowledge: treatment regimen	

other? For example, what is the relationship between pain and mobility? One could reason that increased pain leads to decreased mobility. Here are some other self-talk prompts that support reasoning about Mr. Johnson's nursing care needs. Pain is negatively related to mobility because when there is an increase in pain there is a decrease in mobility. Since mobility is related to active joint movement, this means the greater the pain the greater the restriction of joint movement. The nurse can engage each diagnosis or nursing care need in a similar manner and think about relationships among them using self-talk learning prompts. See Figure 2 for CRW for Mr. Johnson's case.

Iterative reflection, or self-talk of the type illustrated above, sets the stage for weaving a clinical reasoning web. As one continues to think out loud or engage in explanatory self-talk, one begins to see a pattern emerging. Concurrent and iterative reflections and explanations illustrate relationships among keystone issues. In Mr. Johnson's case, these are pain, fatigue, and impaired physical mobility. Relationships among these keystone issues suggest theoretical propositions about how each issue affects the others. A major and significant keystone issue for Mr. Johnson is pain, as it can be hypothesized that pain is the root cause of fatigue and impaired physical mobility. Once we have arrived at a conception of the problem, how does one think clinically about the desired outcome? It is helpful to go back to Kelso's and Engstrom's[15] work on the nature of complementary pairs. The complementary pair is pain ~ comfort.

Such complementary thinking requires creative thinking and is supported by the juxtaposition of the specified present state with the desired opposite or complementary outcome state. Contrasting present state conditions with specified outcome states requires attention and appreciation for understanding the tension between opposites and the complementary nature of outcomes ~ problems. Table 1 compares and contrasts two frames: problem-oriented or outcome-oriented for Mr. Johnson's case.

On one hand, we have reasoning about the problems—that as pain increases so does fatigue, activity intolerance, and impaired physical mobility. On the other hand, we have increasing comfort and pain control which is likely to promote active joint movement, ambulation, and energy endurance. Use of a Clinical Reasoning Web (CRW) helps the nurse visualize relationships and develop propositions about how patient care needs are related. These propositions help to organize and make explicit present states and desired outcomes. The nurse then identifies nursing interventions, activities, and outcome indicators for Mr. Johnson, thus linking the reasoning and explanations of how his nursing care needs or diagnoses interact with each other as a way to represent and frame nursing care issues. By weaving a web of relationships among identified nursing diagnoses associated with a medical condition, the nurse uses thinking strategies to analyze and synthesize functional relationships among diagnostic hypotheses associated with a client's health status. Note that the patients and their primary medical diagnoses are in the center of the web, and the relevant nursing diagnoses are around the edges. Lines of relationship, connection, or association are drawn among the nursing diagnoses. Unidirectional and bidirectional arrows indicate the nonlinear relationships, influences, and effects within the web. Keystone issues become obvious when analyzing the patterns of relationships among the elements of the web and are highlighted with a star.

Nursing Outcomes, Interventions, and Judgments

In considering interventions for Mr. Johnson or another patient, the nurse can turn to the knowledge representations categorized and classified in the Nursing Interventions Classification System (NIC). For example, there are forty-three activities identified for the NIC Intervention for Pain Management. Some include: comprehensive assessment, observing non-verbal cues of discomfort, exploring the patient's knowledge and beliefs about pain, teaching principles of pain management, controlling the environment, and providing optimal pain relief with prescribed analgesics. These activities are in the service of the knowledge representation and defined outcome of comfort. The Nursing Outcomes Classification (NOC) definition of comfort is: extent of positive perception of physical and psychological ease. It can be found at: *http://www.nursing.uiowa.edu/excellence/ nursing_knowledge/clinical_effectiveness/index.htm.*

The following clinical indicators provide ways to measure outcome achievement in the context of a target rating: reported physical well being, symptom control, psychological wellbeing, and pain control. Decision making now becomes the choice of an intervention that supports transitions from present to desired outcomes states. As we choose and act, we are in the process of testing. Testing is defined as thinking about present state transitions to outcome state targets.

Judgments are derived from "tests." Judgments in the OPT model are derived from the four Cs: *Contrast* of present states and desired states; *Criteria* – evidence, clinical indicators, rating scales, and target ratings; *Concurrent thinking* about the effect of the intervention on the identified problem ~ outcomes pair, and *Conclusions* about outcome achievement that can be categorized as, "Yes, the outcome ratings and targets are achieved." Another possible consequence of a judgment is, "No, the ratings and targets have not been achieved." If the targets have not been achieved, the nurse is prompted to think again, reflect, and reframe the issue as it may have transformed into another issue that needs attention.

Obviously, this type of reasoning happens in nanoseconds for experienced clinicians because neural networks and past experiences have added to their knowledge and ability to understand the gestalt, the figure, and ground of such stories quite quickly. The ability to do this type of thinking is a challenge for a novice, and educators and staff development personnel are challenged to make the invisible thinking embedded in this reasoning more visible. Slowing thinking down and making the tacit thinking explicit thinking help novices and students develop the habits of mind and acquire clinical reasoning skill sets. The acquisition of such skills sets requires several types of thinking.

The Thinking that Supports Clinical Reasoning

In the OPT model, the thinking that is involved in clinical reasoning is characterized as:

- Cognitive – Critical thinking

- Metacognitive – Reflective thinking

- Creative – Thinking about the tension between the complementary pairs of present state ~ outcome state

- Systems – The thinking and reasoning about balancing and reinforcing causal loops in a system dynamic

- Complex – The thinking that involves attention to the recursive, nonlinear pattern recognition associated with the identification and creation of clinical reasoning webs, patient care needs, and nursing care responses.

Perkins and Tishman[31] argue there is a need to expand our language about thinking processes and thinking states. They suggest there are "differences that make a difference" in our concept of thinking. For example, they propose language to differentiate the processes, products, stances, and states associated with thinking. For example, thinking processes are "languaged" through such terms as examine, justify, elaborate, reflect, and infer. Thinking products are categorized as a theory, hypothesis, summary, deduction, or guess. Thinking stances are described as agreements, disagreements, questions, concurrence, doubts, or disputes. Thinking states can be defined as confusion, awe, wonder, or being overwhelmed. Educators seldom make explicit the metacognitive nature of thinking and learning involved in clinical reasoning. We seldom take into account the complexity of relationship issues associated with thinking about a patient's needs, given the cast of providers that often represent and frame the care issues differently.

Critical Thinking Supports Clinical Reasoning

Scheffer & Rubenfeld[19] published results of a Delphi study to derive a consensus statement on the nature of critical thinking in nursing. An international panel of expert nurses from nine countries, including Brazil, Canada, England, Iceland, Japan, Korea, Netherlands, Thailand, and twenty-three U.S. states participated in this study between 1995 and 1998. The panel identified and defined ten habits of the mind (affective components) and seven skills (cognitive components) of critical thinking in nursing. The habits of the mind included: confidence, contextual perspective, creativity, flexibility, inquisitiveness, intellectual integrity, intuition, open-mindedness, perseverance, and reflection. Skills of critical thinking in nursing included: analyzing, applying standards, discriminating, information seeking, logical reasoning, and predicting and transforming knowledge. The consensus statement on critical thinking describes critical thinking in nursing as "an essential component of professional accountability and quality nursing care. Critical thinkers in nursing exhibit these habits of the mind: confidence, contextual perspective, creativity, flexibility, inquisitiveness, intellectual integrity, intuition, open-mindedness, perseverance, and reflection. Critical thinkers in nursing practice the cognitive skills of analyzing, applying standards, discriminating, information seeking, logical reasoning, predicting, and transforming knowledge."[19] While critical thinking is a valuable tool in the acquisition of effective reasoning, there are other thinking skills that are perhaps even more important than critical thinking that support the acquisition of clinical reasoning expertise. These are the skills of metacognitive thinking, creative thinking, systems thinking, and complexity thinking.

Creative Thinking Supports Clinical Reasoning

Creative thinking is a requisite metacognitive skill that supports clinical reasoning. It generates novel and useful associations, attributes, elements, images, and abstract relations or sets of operations that better solve a problem, produce a plan, or result in a pattern, structure, or product not clearly present before.[32] Metacognitive knowledge consists primarily of knowledge about what factors or variables act and interact in what ways to affect the course and outcome of cognitive enterprises.[33] It is one's metacognitive knowledge that leads one to select, evaluate, revise, or abandon a line of thinking. Kuiper and Pesut[28] have expanded notions about the relationships between cognition and metacognition relative to clinical reasoning skill acquisition.

Systems and Complexity Thinking
Supports Clinical Reasoning

Two additional types of thinking skills required for effective clinical reasoning are systems thinking and understanding complexity principles. The Clinical Reasoning Web used to support learning of the OPT model is a teaching strategy that supports the development of these skills. According to Senge,[34] systems thinking is a framework that allows one to focus on relationships and patterns rather than objects. Systems thinking encompasses a number of methods, tools, and principles oriented to the

Box 2: Systems thinking description

Systems thinking is a discipline for seeing wholes. It is a framework for seeing interrelationships rather than things, for seeing patterns of change rather than static "snapshots." It is a set of principles, distilled over the course of the twentieth century, spanning fields as diverse as the physical and social sciences, engineering and management....systems thinking is a sensibility for the subtle interconnectedness that gives living systems their unique character.[34] ■

examination and explanation of the interrelationships of variables or forces as part of a common process. Systems thinking makes explicit both the visible and invisible relationships among variables in a system dynamic. Gaining insights into the whole by understanding the linkages and interactions among the elements that comprise the whole "system" is consistent with systems philosophy. It recognizes that all human activity systems are open systems; therefore, they are affected by the environment in which they exist.

Traditional decision making tends to involve linear cause and effect relationships. By taking a systems approach, we can see the whole complex of bidirectional interrelationships. Instead of analyzing a problem in terms of an input and an output, for example, we look at the whole system of inputs, processes, outputs, feedback, and control. This larger picture will typically provide more useful results than traditional methods

It is the use of a CRW that helps illustrate relationships among diagnoses given a particular client story. Systems thinking helps to reveal reinforcing loops, balancing loops, and delays to system dynamics. Consider the interactions and inter-relationships among the four variables of pain, anxiety, energy management, and self care for a patient. How are patterns among these variables mapped, explained, and described? As anxiety increases, does pain increase, and if so, how specifically does the increased pain influence and affect energy management and self care? A systems thinking approach helps address these questions. Refer to Box 2 for further explanation of systems thinking.

Complexity thinking has emerged as an explanatory model for a variety of phenomena. Complexity thinking involves attention to the recursive, nonlinear pattern recognition associated with the identification and creation of clinical reasoning webs, patient care needs, and nursing care responses. Complexity thinking supports reasoning as one considers the multiple interactions of various elements in a given situation.. In patient care situations, complexity thinking involves attention to the medical diagnosis and physician framing of the situation as well as the system of the family, the nursing care needs, and any other number of disciplines that may be involved in a patient's care. Using Glouberman and Zimmerman's[35] conceptualization of simple, complicated, and complex as described in the Chapter by Lindberg and Lindberg, an example of something simple in terms of clinical reasoning would be following a standard assessment checklist or form. Something complicated would be crafting or formulating a nursing diagnosis from cues and inferences, and something complex would be the process of considering the patient's story as a whole and ex-

Box 3: Twenty questions that OPTimize care

1. Tell me the story.
2. How are you framing the situation?
3. What diagnoses have you generated?
4. What outcomes do you have in mind given the diagnoses?
5. What evidence supports those diagnoses?
6. How does a reasoning web reveal relationships among the identified problems (diagnoses)?
7. What keystone issue(s) emerge?
8. How is the present state defined?
9. What are the desired outcomes?
10. What are the gaps or complementary pairs (~) of outcomes and present states?
11. What are the clinical indicators of the desired outcomes?
12. On what scales will the desired outcomes be rated?
13. How will you know when the desired targeted outcomes are achieved?
14. What clinical decisions or interventions help to achieve the outcomes?
15. What specific intervention activities will you implement?
16. Why are you considering these activities?
17. How are you defining your testing (concurrent thinking and consideration about present state transitions to outcome state targets) in this particular case?
18. Given your testing, what is your clinical judgment?
19. Based on your judgment, have you achieved the outcome or do you need to reframe the situation?
20. How specifically will you take this experience and learning with you into future as you reason about similar cases? ■

amining the relationships among care needs, outcomes, interventions, and judgments.

Complexity theory teaches that when our psychological perspective shifts, we experience patterns and relationships in new ways. Small changes can have big effects, and diverse, chaotic systems self-organize around attractors. Complexity thinking helps us master the complexity of clinical reasoning and the complementary nature of paired relationships[15] that sustain outcome ~ problem specification and clinical actions and interventions that lead to judgments about outcome achievements. Given the OPT structure, as well as the teaching and learning strategies associated with the OPT model, clinicians, from a variety of disciplines, may be able to adopt or adapt the model to achieve some of the goals of clinical reasoning. Hopefully, the OPT model will help people understand causality, make multivariate comparisons, examine relevant evidence, and assess the credibility of evidence and conclusions as they reason about complex patient care problems.

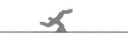

Complexity theory teaches that when our psychological perspective shifts, we experience patterns and relationships in new ways.

Twenty Questions That "OPTimize" Care

The twenty questions in Box 3 help to summarize the art, science, and complexity of clinical reasoning. Using the OPT model and the CRW along with attention to knowledge representation and framing, it is possible to appreciate the complexity of clinical reasoning.

Reasoning into the Future
through the Knowledge Work of Informatics

Pesut and Herman[23] have written about the evolution and development of the nursing process in the United States, identifying the following three generations of nursing process:

* 1950-1970 – Problems to process

- 1970-1990 – Diagnosis and reasoning

- 1990-present – Outcome specification and testing

As knowledge representation schemes and discipline-specific framing evolve, the nursing profession is likely to see future transformations of the nursing process. The development of integrated sets of nursing diagnoses, interventions, and outcomes will emerge as we continue to push the frontiers of data mining using the information and nursing informatics systems that are now being built. The future may witness developments in data mining and knowledge modeling and building, along with the development of models or archetypes of care, that can be used to predict care needs based on evidence and modeling techniques. In order to more systematically and intentionally refine our models of care based on informatics, healthcare cultures need to value nursing knowledge representation and framing. Nurses need to embrace knowledge work as a professional responsibility and appreciate the complexity of clinical reasoning. The profession needs leadership for change that supports complexity thinking as well as models and methods that embrace innovation, creativity, and complexity.

A Bridge to the Future of Clinical Reasoning: Reflections from the Edge

By editors Curt Lindberg & Claire Lindberg

This book is essentially about evolution—a developing young science and the implications it holds for nursing practice, leadership, teaching, and research. Since it is about evolution, little is settled and new insights and possibilities are constantly emerging. As such, this book seeks to go beyond presentation of the current state of Complexity Science in nursing by pointing out possible avenues for future development and by stimulating conversations within the nursing community and between nurses and complexity scientists in the hope that they trigger new advances.

This chapter illuminates how thinking about clinical reasoning has evolved and is continuing to evolve in relation to discoveries in science and nursing. We will thus use this opportunity to engage in a conversation with this chapter to highlight this movement and spark conversations about possible future directions for Complexity Science-informed approaches to clinical reasoning.

The OPT model can be seen as a bridge that transcends and includes conventional first and second generation nursing decision making models, such as APIE and ADPIE. These more traditional models were grounded in linear and reductionist problem solving models in contrast to more systems thinking and dynamic frameworks. The OPT model opens the door to the domain of Complexity Science-inspired clinical decision making. There are aspects of the model that reflect some complexity principles. From a Complexity Science perspective, the following stand out:

- The model makes explicit the complex nature of clinical reasoning and emphasizes the importance of iterative reflection as a key to learning, decision making, and action. Complexity Science points our attention to the central role played by interaction in shaping patterns of behavior in systems. Ongoing reflections are, in essence, interactions between one's experiences and ways of making sense of experience. Iteration is a route to emergence and learning.

- The OPT model encourages nurses to seek stories from patients. Complexity scientists would likely view narratives as better vehicles for capturing the intricacies and nuances of human experience than asking closed-ended questions or using checklists or printed history forms. Stories reflect the unique and complex nature of the lives of patients.

- Creative thinking as developed in the OPT model reminds us of the central complexity concepts of self-organization and emergence.

- The OPT model implicitly acknowledges the nonlinear nature of problem solving and nurses' clinical decision making. As such, the OPT model recognizes the complex nature of the interactions that take place within the patient and between the patient and the nurse.

- In recognizing that the nurse must constantly assess and reassess the patient and repeatedly shift gears as the patient responds to interventions or as the patient's care needs change, the OPT model acknowledges that prediction is limited and control is not possible. This is in keeping with the Complexity Science understanding of the nature of change and the impossibility of anticipating future behavior in complex adaptive systems.

We note however, some challenges and limitations to the model based on our understanding of Complexity Science. The following observations about the OPT model are not meant to convey that the OPT model and its predecessors do not have value. On the contrary, many views of Complexity Science would suggest they are very appropriate in certain circumstances, particularly those patient care issues that fall into the categorizations of simple or complicated as described by Glouberman and Zimmerman.[35] (See Chapter by Lindberg and Lindberg for a further explanation of Glouberman and Zimmerman's framework). It is when the nurse is faced with the most complex patients or patient care problems that the model proves insufficient. There are very complex patients whose conditions may be challenging to analyze using this model. Examples include patients with multiple, interacting conditions or care issues, patients with very unstable medical conditions, frail elderly patients, patients with volatile psychiatric conditions, patients with difficult family situations, or those without identifiable family or community support. In such cases, a more complex model may be needed.

- Complexity Science notes that any system, human or otherwise, is composed of multiple interacting agents, and that even the smallest change by one of the agents may have large effects on the system. This property of unpredictability calls into question the practicality of identifying one or a few keystone issues as the focus of intervention. Indeed, in some very complex cases, identifying a keystone issue or a few such issues and focusing action on those issues may obscure other critical areas where nursing intervention is needed.

- The OPT model focuses on clinical reasoning by one nurse about one patient. This focus has its utility, particularly regarding education of nursing students and novice nurses. However, in reality, no nurse-patient dyad exists in isolation. One of the strongest influences on the interactions between the nurse and patient is the family. Hartwick Doane, and Varcoe state that "nothing exists independent of its relationship to something or someone else,"[36] and that those relationship connections and past experiences impact every aspect of the nurse-patient relationship. Most patients have strong and enduring relationships with family members and have had experiences that affect their interpretations of events, their thinking and their behavior. An example of a model that incorporates family is advanced by Lannaman, Harris, Bakos, and Baker[37] in their writing on end of life care. These authors suggest that clinicians use their power to "write a prescription" for family conversations to aid patients, loved ones, and clinicians in moving from extended, and many times fruitless, efforts to cure cancer patients to conversations about palliative care. The clinician then joins the conversation not as the expert but as another voice. Two new actions are contained in this strategy—the recommendation for widening the conversation and a shift in the role and power position of the clinician. Both are designed to change the pattern of relating with patients and families and to create more effective paths forward. Such family-centered thinking should be factored into our decision making and clinical reasoning models as they advance.

- Diversity is another important concept in Complexity Science. While the OPT model is useful in helping nursing students and other novices work through a patient care problem by themselves, this does not fully reflect the reality of healthcare. In almost every healthcare situation, the nurse acts in collaboration with, not in isolation from, other healthcare professionals. The interdisciplinary nature of care is an area where further development of the model can and should occur.

The OPT model has had tremendous influence in the nursing community, particularly in nursing education. It is expected it will continue to do so. As such, we present the above not to diminish the importance of the ideas within the model but with the hope of stimulating conversations within the nursing community that contribute to expansion of the OPT model into the next generation of clinical reasoning.

Daniel Pesut, PhD PMHCNS-BC, FAAN, is professor and associate dean for graduate programs at Indiana University School of Nursing and has more than thirty-five years of experience in nursing practice, education, administration, and research. Dr. Pesut is a board certified advanced practice registered nurse in adult psychiatric-mental health nursing. He has held both academic and nursing service positions and has gained insights and understanding from his experiences as a staff nurse, clinical nurse specialist, faculty member, and director of nursing services, associate dean, department chair, consultant, therapist, and trainer. Dr. Pesut serves on the Board of Trustees of Plexus Institute.

Works Cited

1. K. Lewin, *Field Theory in Social Sciences: Selected Theoretical Papers by Kurt Lewin* (London: Tavistock, 1952), 169.

2. E. Tufte, *Beautiful Evidence* (Chesire: Graphic Press, 2006).

3. Kaufman et al., "Frames, Framing and Reframing," 2006. Available from http://crinfo.beyondintractability.org/essay/faming.

4. R. Davis, H. Shrobe, and P. Szolovits, "What Is Knowledge Representation," *AI Magazine* 14, no. 1 (1993): 17-33, 21.

5. L. Taylor and W. Care, "Nursing Education As Cognitive Apprenticeship: A Framework for Clinical Education," *Nurse Educator* 24, no. 4 (1999): 31-36.

6. North American Nursing Diagnosis Association, *Nursing Diagnoses: Definitions and Classifications 2004-2006* (Philadelphia: NANDA, 2005).

7. J. Dochterman and D. Jones, *Unifying Nursing Languages: The Harmonization of NANDA, NIC and NOC* (Silver Spring: American Nurses Association, 2003).

8. M. Blegen and T. Tripp-Reiner, "Implications of Nursing Taxonomies for Middle-Range Theory Development," *Advances in Nursing Science* 19, no. 3 (1998): 37-49.

9. D. J. Pesut, "Nursing Nomenclatures and Eye-Roll Anxiety Control," *Journal of Professional Nursing* 18, no. 1 (2002): 3-4.

10. D. J. Pesut, "21st Century Nursing Knowledge Work: Reasoning into the Future," in *Nursing and Informatics for the 21st Century: An International Look at Practice Trends and the Future*, ed. C. Weaver et al. (Chicago: Health Care Information and Management Systems Society, 2006), 13-23.

11. American Nurses Association, *Nursing a Social Policy Statement* (Washington, D.C.: American Nurses Association, 1980), 9.

12. C. Pedon-McAlpine, "Expert Thinking in Nursing Practice: Implications for Supporting Expertise," *Nursing and Health Sciences* 1 (1999): 131-137.

13. P. Benner, P. Hopper-Kyriakidis, and D. Stannard, *Clinical Wisdom and Interventions in Critical Care: A Thinking-In-Action Approach* (Philadelphia: W.B. Saunders, 1999).

14. P. Benner, C. Tanner, and C. Chesla, *Expertise in Nursing Practice* (New York: Springer Publishing Company, 1997).

15. J. Kelso and D. Engstrom, *The Complementary Nature* (Cambridge: A Bradford Book, 2006).

16. N. Facione and P. Facione, "Externalizing the Critical Thinking in Knowledge Development and Clinical Judgment," *Nursing Outlook* 44, no. 3 (1996): 129-136.

17. K. Bowles, "Research Briefs: The Relationship of Critical-Thinking Skills and the Clinical-Judgement Skills of Baccalaureate Nursing Students," *Journal of Nursing Education* 39, no. 8 (2000): 373-376.

18. F. D. Hicks, "Critical Thinking: Toward a Nursing Science Perspective," *Nursing Science Quarterly* 14, no. 1 (2001): 14-21.

19. B. Scheffer and G. Rubenfeld, "A Consensus Statement on Critical Thinking in Nursing," *Journal of Nursing Education* 39, no. 8 (2000): 352-359, 356.

20. S. Burns and C. Bulman, *Reflective Practice in Nursing: The Growth of the Professional Practitioner* 2nd ed. (London: Blackwell Science, 2000).

21. C. Johns, *Becoming a Reflective Practitioner* (London: Blackwell Science, 2000).

22. M. Johnson and others, *Nursing Diagnoses, Outcomes, and Interventions: NANDA, NOC, and NIC Linkages* (St. Louis: C.V. Mosby, 2001).

23. D. Pesut and J. Herman, "OPT: Transformation of the Nursing Process for Contemporary Practice," *Nursing Outlook* 46 (1998): 29-36.

24. D. Pesut and J. Herman, *Clinical Reasoning: The Art and Science of Critical and Creative Thinking* (New York: Delmar Publishers, 1999).

25. American Nurses Association, *Nursing: Scope and Standards of Practice* (Washington, D.C.: ANA Publishing, 2004).

26. D. J. Pesut, "Clinical Judgement: Foreground/Background," *Journal of Professional Nursing* 17, no. 5 (2001): 215.

27. D. Pesut, "Toward the Future," in *Nursing in Contemporary Society: Issues, Trends, and Transitions to Practice*, ed. L. Haynes, H. Butcher, and T. Boese. (Upper Saddle River: Prentice Hall, 2004).

28. R. Kuiper and D. Pesut, "Promoting Cognitive and Metacognitive Reflective Learning Skills in Nursing Practice: Self-Regulated Learning Theory," *Journal of Advanced Nursing* 45, no. 4 (2004): 381-391.

29. G. Klein, *Sources of Power: How People Make Decisions* (Cambridge: MIT Press, 1999).

30. A. L. Barabasi, *Linked: The New Science of Networks* (Cambridge: Perseus, 2002), 43.

31. D. N. Perkins, E. Jay, and S. Tishman, "New Conceptions of Thinking From Ontology to Education," *Educational Psychologist* 28, no. 1 (1993): 67-85.

32. D. Pesut, "Toward a New Definition of Creativity," *Nurse Educator* 10, no. 1 (1985): 5.

33. J. Flavell, "Metacognition and Cognitive Monitoring: A New Area of Cognitive-Developmental Inquiry," *American Psychologist* 34 (1979): 906-911.

34. P. Senge, *The Fifth Discipline: The Art and Practice of the Learning Organization* (New York: Doubleday Currency, 1990).

35. S. Glouberman and B. Zimmerman, "Complicated and Complex Systems: What Would Successful Reform of Medicare Look Like?," 2007. Available from http://www.change-ability.ca/publications.html.

36. G. Hartick Doane and C. Varcoe, *Family Nursing as Relational Inquiry: Developing Health-promoting Practice* (Philadelphia: Lippincott, Williams & Wilkins, 2005), 52.

37. J.W. Lannamann et al., "Ending the End-of-Life Communication Impasse: A Dialogic Intervention," in *Cancer Communication in Aging*, ed. L. Sparks, D. O'Hair, and G. Kreps. (Cresskill: Hampton Press, Forthcoming).

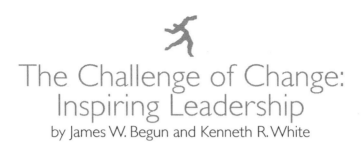

The Challenge of Change: Inspiring Leadership
by James W. Begun and Kenneth R. White

I suspect that the fate of all complex adapting systems in the biosphere – from single cells to economies – is to evolve to a natural state between order and chaos, a grand compromise between structure and surprise.[1]

The need to adapt to a changing environment characterizes all living systems. As the healthcare system evolves in complexity and direction, it is incumbent on those intent on leading the system to change as well, and to develop new and more powerful means of leadership. Such leadership requires an appreciation for the complexity of the healthcare system.

The complexity of the healthcare system, described in detail in Wiggins' chapter, serves as both a challenge and an opportunity for leadership by individual nurses and their organizations and associations. For some, the high level of change and complexity is overwhelming, frustrating, and disempowering. For others, understanding and learning about the complex world of healthcare can energize and empower them to incredible accomplishments. It is the goal of this chapter to contribute to such an understanding and to expand the energy and power of the community of nursing in the healthcare system.

The focus of this chapter is on nurses, nursing organizations, and nursing associations in their leadership roles and activities. The meaning of leadership from a Complexity Science perspective is developed first. Drawing on the work of Drath,[2-4] leadership under conditions of complexity, there are three key competencies essential to meeting complex challenges— shared sensemaking, exploring, and connecting. Individuals, groups, associations, and organizations of all types within the nursing community accomplish leadership activities. Box 1 includes definitions of these three competencies.

Leadership arises to accomplish three important tasks that are faced by human systems: providing direction, inspiring commitment, and facing adaptive challenges.

The assets of the nursing community are assessed in relation to the accomplishment of these three competencies. Opportunities to accomplish shared sensemaking, exploring, and connecting within nursing are noted, and the chapter ends by commenting on nursing's potential contributions to leadership in the larger healthcare system.

Complexity-Informed Leadership Includes Everyone

Leadership arises to accomplish three important tasks that are faced by human systems: providing direction, inspiring commitment, and facing adaptive challenges.[4] Direction involves the articulation of mission, vision, and strategies that identify a destination and a path toward it. Inspiring commitment involves developing cohesion so that members or units of a system can work together. Adaptive challenges cause confusion to system members, and facing those challenges requires developing a sense of what the challenge is, and what it means. All three tasks are critical to the sustenance of human systems.

Theoretically, in a simple and hierarchical organization or community, these leadership tasks can be readily accomplished by individuals in positions of formal authority. Leadership can be a personal or an individual activity, and followers can abrogate key decision-making activities to the leader. In a more complicated setting, leaders need to influence others so that the system as a whole can work toward the same tasks of direction, inspiration, and facing challenges. Leadership is interpersonal, and the person who has the most influence becomes the leader. In even more complex settings, accomplishing the tasks of leadership requires leaders to facilitate a process whereby members or units of the system construct direction themselves, build their own commitment, and confront and overcome complex challenges together. Leadership becomes collaborative and facilitative. It becomes the responsibility of everyone, and the tasks of leadership are realized through emergent, relational dialogue among diverse individuals and organizations. It is this concept of leadership that is most difficult to attain, yet most necessary for complex systems to adopt and sustain.

Box 1: Leadership competencies: sensemaking, exploring, and connecting

- **Sensemaking:** The term sensemaking, coined by organizational behavior scholar, Karl E. Weick, refers to a developing set of ideas with explanatory possibilities rather than a body of knowledge. Weick maintains knowledge is a socially constructed understanding through which we make sense of our circumstances. Sensemaking should be distinguished from interpretation. Sensemaking is always about an activity or a process in which an individual is engaged and making a contribution, while interpretation is apt to be a product, or the discovery of something waiting to be uncovered. According to Weick, sensemaking requires us to generate understanding by looking at the interactions among people, their ideas and their points of view.[38]

- **Exploration:** This competency reflects the search for individual career and workplace choices, for new roles and opportunities, and for new directions in practice and education that provide the knowledge necessary for growth and change.

- **Connecting:** The term connecting refers to the multiple ways nurses and nursing organizations establish relationships with and build networks among patients, families, communities and other healthcare professionals and organizations. An important role of nurses today is to ensure patient safety by acting as the hub of the interdisciplinary healthcare team. ■

Traditional approaches to leadership have emphasized the personal and interpersonal perspectives on leadership, and perhaps those were appropriate for understanding and action in simple and complicated systems. But as Complexity Science informs, the work world is more often complex than simple or complicated (see Chapter 2 by Lindberg & Lindberg for further discussion). The important challenges to individuals and organizations are confusing rather than clear, and the future is murky and uncertain. A complexity-informed view of leadership is necessary to help us effectively explore and live in this world.

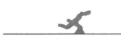

In the traditional vein, leaders are individuals who perform relatively public, heroic acts to create major transformations. This perspective neglects the acts of individuals whose less visible, cumulative, day-to-day, incremental actions spark transformative change when combined with similar acts of others, whether or not any of the individuals are in positions of formal authority.

Nurses and nursing organizations function in a complex world. Hierarchies and guidelines exist, but are not sufficient to accomplish the work of clinical nurses or the work of nursing organizations. Clinical work requires that nurses integrate resources from a variety of sources, for example, information technology, patients and families, dietary, and pharmacy. Clinical nurses face complexity every day in their multiple and diverse functions as patient care providers, case managers, administrators, patient and family educators, quality managers, and so on. The same degree of complexity is true for nursing roles in administration, education, and other settings.

At the collective level of the nursing profession, complexity is equally obvious. Decisions about creating new degrees and specialties, about the role of the professional association, and about effecting improvement in working conditions are highly complex. Such conditions cry out for leadership that is, in the words of Raelin,[5;6] collective, compassionate, concurrent, and collaborative.

A complexity-informed approach to leadership is more useful than a traditional approach in helping individuals and organizations make positive change in complex systems. As noted earlier, leadership traditionally has been viewed as an attribute of individuals, particularly of individuals who are in strong positions of authority in organizations, associations, and other social systems. In the traditional vein, leaders are individuals who perform relatively public, heroic acts to create major transformations. This perspective neglects the acts of individuals whose less visible, cumulative, day-to-day, incremental actions spark transformative change when combined with similar acts of others, whether or not any of the individuals are in positions of formal authority. The traditional conceptualization ignores the nonlinear nature of change in complex systems. Small actions can have huge effects in complex systems through reverberations via connections among the units in the systems. Transformative change can occur through the "small" actions of "small" individuals and other units in systems if those actions are undertaken in the right place, at the right time.

In addition, the traditional approach to leadership and change conceives leadership largely as a top-down activity. For example, perhaps the most popular model of organizational change is Kotter's eight-step model.[7:7] The model promotes creating a sense of urgency in the organization, building a leadership coalition for change, and implementing a series of executive decisions to create conditions receptive to change. All of these steps largely assume that successful change requires top leadership participation and direction. This model is directly challenged by the reality of change in complex systems.[8] Successful change can emerge from anywhere in complex systems—from the bottom, middle, or top. In other words, all complex systems can produce change, by self-organizing.

The traditional approach to leadership, with its focus on individuals, also neglects the collective acts of teams, organizations, associations, and other social systems as a whole. Leadership activities may emerge from the work of multiple individuals in multiple social systems, with none of the individuals particularly serving in a traditional role of leader. For example, the way that a group of nurses implements a new care process in a hospital unit contributes to leadership. Their actions both influence and reflect the community of nursing's direction, commitment, and adaptation to challenges. In this sense, one can identify social systems that perform leadership activities, and refer to teams, organizations, and associations, as well as individuals, as "leaders" in a social system.

This chapter focuses on nurses at the registered nurse level and beyond, including staff nurses, nurse practitioners (NPs), nurse midwives, nurse anesthetists, Clinical Nurse Leaders (CNLs®), and clinical nurse specialists. These clinical practitioners are supported by nurse administrators, educators, and researchers, who are part of the nursing community. Organizations and associations that represent individual members of the community also comprise the professional nursing community.

Leadership in Complex Systems: Sensemaking, Connecting, and Exploring

As proposed above, leadership is a process that is used to accomplish a set of key tasks in human systems: providing direction, inspiring commitment, and facing adaptive challenges. In complex systems, these tasks are addressed through three competencies: shared sensemaking, exploring, and connecting. The three leadership competencies are interdependent, and activities can overlap the three categories, but the categories are useful for understanding and shaping leadership activity. The leadership competencies can be performed by individuals, groups, teams, organizations, and associations in the community of practice.

The first complexity leadership competency is shared sensemaking. Complex or adaptive challenges, such as those faced both within nursing and within the healthcare system, do not have obvious solutions. Drath[3] points out that complex challenges "cause confusion, ambiguity, conflict, and stress." Shared sensemaking allows participants to understand the nature of problems and opportunities, and to be able to propose innovative solutions. Competent leaders and leading organizations collaboratively work with their teams, groups, and peer organizations to interpret the meaning of their work. In doing so, they develop a sense of identity, pride, and commitment to their communities.

Second, facing complexity involves making choices and learning about complex challenges through action. This is done through exploration. Exploration requires bold decisions and execution. Leaders focus on the choices to be made in response to questions including: Where are we going? What will we become and do in the future? How will we get there?[4] Most often, decisions are not black-and-white or clear-cut, but rather gray. Learning about the world requires taking action and learning from those actions. This leadership competency requires a level of comfort with decision making under uncertainty, and a commitment to flexibility, risk taking, and learning.

Finally, complex challenges require "people and organizations to develop and enrich their forms of connection."[3] Connections between individuals, groups, teams, functions, and organizations are all necessary to share issues, insights, fears, dreams, innovations, and creativity. Complex challenges alter existing connections and create new ones. The introduction of a new nursing role in the workplace, for example, the CNL role, creates a new pattern of connections for all those in the setting. The ability to develop new relationships among individuals, groups, and organizations is a competency of leadership under conditions of complexity.

Taken together, these three competencies enable agents in a complex system to exert some proactive influence over their emergent future. In facing complex challenges, leadership is not an individual task. Exploring, making sense, and connecting cannot be taken on by individuals in isolation. They all involve consulting and learning from others. For example, providing excellent care to a chronic care patient (at the individual nurse level) or developing chronic care guidelines (at an organizational level) are complex challenges. Providing excellent care may entail relationships with the patient and his or her social system members, and other professionals from functions and disciplines such as physical therapy, pharmacy, pastoral care, social work, nutrition, administration, and finance. People, groups, and organizations from diverse circumstances are needed to provide leadership in the form of sensemaking, exploring, and connecting.

Complexity Leadership in Nursing: An Asset Inventory

Leadership tasks in systems are not undertaken in a vacuum. As individuals think about how to accomplish the leadership tasks of shared sensemaking, exploring, and connecting, they need to be aware of the opportunities before them. An aid in doing so is to conduct an inventory of assets of the system. What system assets can contribute to more effective sensemaking, exploring, and connecting? Often these assets are overlooked because of the focus of leaders on problem solving rather than opportunity generation. An asset-based or appreciative inquiry approach to change can energize and empower commitment and innovation in ways that a problem solving approach cannot.[9] An appreciative view of the profession is reflected in the opinion piece, "The Most Modern Profession," reprinted in Box 2, at the end of this chapter.

The professional community of nursing has a powerful arsenal of assets. These assets are particularly valuable as nursing undertakes a stronger leadership role in the healthcare system. The community of nursing is endowed with particular advantages as it explores and connects to the larger healthcare system and performs other leadership activities. These assets are discussed below.

Size and Scope

First, the nursing community is huge in size, and its reach across healthcare delivery settings and specialties is extremely broad. As a social system, nursing is the both the largest and the most complex of the health professions. Nursing constitutes more than twenty-five percent of the U.S. workforce.[10] The vast size (some two million registered nurses alone) of nursing in the United States compares to the approximately 600,000 physicians, 170,000 pharmacists, and 150,000 dentists. Nursing is highly differentiated internally, divided not only by level of training and clinical specialty, but also practice setting. Almost one hundred associations at the national level, and many more at the state level, populate the organizational field of nursing.[11]

Stable and High Demand for Services

Second, services offered by nursing are periodically in undersupply. The supply of registered nurses is projected to be some twenty percent below demand by the year 2020, as the aging workforce retires and younger cohorts turn to other types of work.[12] While there are negative consequences of undersupply, it puts nurses in a stronger bargaining position with employer organizations. It also ensures that nursing will remain one of the careers most recommended to individuals entering the labor force.

While inpatient staff nurse jobs may decline, the expansion of home and outpatient therapies and other new therapies has created new job markets for nurses.[13] The growth of outpatient care has opened more opportunities for nursing roles in home care, assisted care, and other ambulatory settings, while the aging of the population adds to chronic care needs and geriatric care needs, both of which nursing is poised to address. The rise of the more educated and more demanding consumer opens new opportunities for nurses to meet demands for accessible, high-quality care. One result of this is that NPs are increasingly finding their niche in primary care settings, including both clinics and private practices. Consumers seem quite accepting of the provision of primary healthcare by nurses.[14] The accelerating demand for complementary and holistic therapies contributes to the demand for nursing services, as nursing's holistic view of the individual is consistent with many complementary therapies. Finally, nurses are positioned to supply the bulk of care for chronic disease management, as the balance between acute and chronic disease increasingly shifts in the direction of chronic disease.

Unparalleled Trust

Third, nursing has earned tremendous respect from the public. Nursing is consistently rated the most trusted occupation in the United States. For example, eighty-four percent of the public in 2006 rated nurses' honesty and ethical standards as high or very high, with pharmacists ranking second at seventy-three percent.[15] Nurses have led this particular list in all but one year since they were first added to the poll in 1999. This level of trust represents a reservoir of goodwill that any business organization would find invaluable. Even more remarkable is that a profession that has been both internally divided and often underappreciated by other clinical disciplines, organizational administration, and payer organizations has achieved this level of trust.

Nurses' Role in the Interdisciplinary Team

Finally, the role of nursing places nurses at the center of interdisciplinary, interprofessional exchange centered on the patient. The individual nurse is the node of a highly complex interchange. Nurses are the nodal point for the delivery of healthcare interventions. They are responsible for screening and assessing the input of the patient and the patient's family. They also must consider the socioeconomic and environmental conditions faced by the patient. Nursing is a health profession that is closely identified with the patient, and in many ways is closest to understanding the patient as a complex, whole person.

At the level of the individual nurse, these assets combine to empower a leadership orientation: Nurses provide a needed service, have a large number of colleagues who share their circumstances, are uniquely appreciated by their clients, and are critical players in the healthcare system. At the collective level, these assets are a strong foundation for group and organizational leadership.

The Emerging Future of Leadership in Nursing

The assets of the professional nursing community can be and are being leveraged to create a more powerful and energizing future for nursing. Shared sensemaking is resulting in a new appreciation for the nursing role. Individual nurses are exploring new, more powerful directions and roles, and connections are expanding in ways that benefit the community of nursing. These changes can be accelerated and deepened depending on the actions and choices of nurses and nursing organizations. To some degree, the future will be determined by choices yet to be made by individuals and organizations within the community of nursing.

This section outlines a vision for a nursing future that builds on an understanding of leadership in complex systems. This interpretation of the future is subjective, of course, and it is intended to focus on the positive. This is not to deny the existence of barriers, such as challenging working conditions in many settings for nurses. The existence of a positive vision for the future is energizing. This is particularly true if nursing is emboldened to use its leadership assets in new ways. The vision can be used to guide individual nurses and their organizations to undertake and achieve leadership in ways they otherwise would not consider. Next, we outline ways in which the nursing community can make sense, explore, and connect in the future.

Shared Sensemaking

How does nursing "make sense" of itself? How do nurses, nursing organizations, and associations interpret and explain the role of nursing in the healthcare system? Historically, dating at least from the influence of Florence Nightingale in the middle and late 1800s,[16] a key theme in nursing's sensemaking has been the concept of caring. Caring is not just a concept that is a value judgment (one cares or does not care), but rather caring in this context means mindful, deliberate presence in order to co-create with the patient a preferred regimen to improve quality of life and to restore a person's wholeness. The concept has been elaborated extensively by nursing theorists.[17;18] Caring has been a characteristic that has been used to keep the nursing community together in order to create cohesion and collective identity.[19]

Today, the nursing community is building on and around its historical focus on caring in several different ways. The appreciation for the historical identity of nursing, coupled with adaptation to a new world, is creating a more powerful core that is better suited to hold together the diverse pieces of nursing.[20-22]

Second, there is growing acceptance of "caring" as a legitimate feature of quality healthcare services, both within and outside nursing. Nurses recognize the integral essence of caring as the focal point of the client-nurse relationship. Nelson and Gordon[23] see a future in which nurses reject the "false polarity" of caring and science, and emphasize "their scientific and medical knowledge, without apology, without it being considered the sign of an 'uncaring' nurse or a wannabe doctor." Caring is seen as consistent with, rather than the opposite of, (or opposed to) scientific knowledge.

Sensemaking enables participants in a complex system to understand and be committed to their roles. Historically, an aspect of nursing's sensemaking has been the notion that nursing has "underdog" status in the healthcare system—that it is under-appreciated and oppressed. This under-appreciation was related to the fact that women largely provided the basic caring function in Western healthcare institutions since the origins of these institutions,[24] to the largely female composition of the nursing community, and to the traditionally passive role expectations of females in society.[25;26] In the past, nursing has been described by Roberts (1983) as exhibiting oppressed group or victim behavior, which has resulted in division and lack of cohesiveness in nursing groups.

For a variety of reasons, the nursing community is moving beyond a posture of victimization to one that is more energizing and positive. Improvements in women's place in the workforce and the declining preponderance of men in the physician and administration workforce are relevant to enhancing the self-identity of nursing. Newer generations of nurses have less concern for history and how nursing once was and older generations are retiring. Nursing is no longer viewed by those entering it as one of a few choices for women (for example, nursing vs. education); they deliberately choose it for job security, income potential, career mobility and variety.

In summation, the nursing community's identity is becoming more complex and more positive. Members of the community are able to respect and use the historical focus on caring but also incorporate science and recognize the need to empirically assess the value of caring. The core concept of caring is being applied in the face of new realities. In the words of McDaniel and Driebe[27] as leaders in a complex world, nurses and nursing organizations are both "remembering (and forgetting) history."

Exploring

Exploration is reflected in the strategic choices individuals and organizations in the community of practice make about careers and about shifting nursing's role in the healthcare system. Exploration possibilities have been constrained by the fact that there are multiple educational pathways to entry-level professional nursing, such as the two-year associate degree, three-year diploma, and baccalaureate degree. Much of professional nursing's exploration energy has been directed at efforts to standardize the entry-level requirement to the baccalaureate degree, with limited success.

During the same period, however, exploration efforts have been successful in producing specialized advanced practice roles for nurses at the master's degree level, for example, clinical nurse specialists (CNSs) and NPs. The two roles are important expansions of the traditional nursing role, as are two other successful advanced practice specialty roles, the certified registered nurse anesthetist (CRNA) and the certified nurse midwife (CNM). There are signs that nursing will continue to explore new opportunities, regardless of internal divisions, or that internal divisions will be resolved. (In Ontario, for example, the baccalaureate-entry level has been accepted through collaborative efforts of nursing organizations.) New roles and credentials include the Doctor of Nursing Practice, a clinically-oriented doctoral degree,[28] and the CNL, discussed below. Both are controversial and may or may not succeed. Regardless, they evidence proactive efforts by segments of nursing to explore, grow, and develop new ways of learning. The community of nursing should be strong enough to not only survive but become stronger through learning from these new developments, whether they become permanent or not.

At the individual level, nurses are making "exploration" choices in new and exciting ways. Some students are entering schools of nursing at an older age and with different backgrounds, as well as different expectations. They often are employed in full-time careers or are raising families.[29] The new entrant may be a second-degree or alternative-pathway student, with a non-nursing background, who is more interested in direct entry to the NP role rather than gaining experience and professional socialization as a staff nurse.[30] Many of the "new" nurses are interested in creating their own practices with well-defined business missions,[31] professional autonomy, and good incomes.[32] Some choose to pursue careers related to but outside of traditional nursing, in areas such as pharmaceutical marketing, child care services, complementary and alternative therapies, and managed care. These developments make nursing an attractive option for a variety of entrants and if pursued, marketed, and celebrated by the community of nursing, will ensure a strong influx of motivated new nurses.

To summarize, nursing continues to upgrade requirements for entry-level and advanced practice and to individually and collectively explore new roles. The hope is that such efforts will not splinter the community. Time will tell if the historical internal schisms will abate, allowing the community to move upward and outward rather than focusing on internal issues. Paradoxically, if such splintering occurs, the outcome might be one of creative new innovations and role emergence. Nursing's exploration activities reveal a greater appreciation for complexity and diversity, and more collective, collaborative leadership.

Connecting

Connecting activities is the third set of complexity leadership competencies. Individuals and organizations create deeper understanding and insight by connecting to others. Historically, at the clinical level, nursing care by definition has involved connection with the patient. In the early and middle 1900s, that connection was based substantially on meeting the comfort care needs of patients, such as changing bed linens, assisting with personal hygiene, medication administration, treatments, and assistance with activities of daily living. Relative to the more modern role of the nurse that has evolved, the connection with the patient in the past was relatively simple. Today, nursing maintains its historical connection to the patient at the clinical level, but it is broadening and deepening that relationship with the patient and family. Connecting to the patient in a more holistic way is a trend that has been underway for many years. The connection includes spiritual and complementary care services that are patient-driven. The nurse's role has evolved to include using the art and science of nursing to connect the right people with the right knowledge in the best interest of the patient. Sometimes this means intervening to obtain medications, to suggest courses of treatment, to recommend community healthcare and social services, or to educate the patient and his or her family about their disease or illness. The nurse is a patient-centered facilitator with a broader array of resources. In this way, nursing's connection to the patient has become deeper and broader. The nurse listens to, interprets, and facilitates responses to the patient's needs by connecting the patient with the relevant professionals, family, and social support network. The nurse is a "specialist" in representing the patient's needs, rather than an outside expert "giving" knowledge to a client.

In addition, nursing's connection with the patient creates more leverage for nursing within delivery organizations. This development has been enabled in part by nursing's own leadership activities, but also by three powerful trends that increase the importance of the nursing role.

First are the findings that healthcare settings have major challenges around quality and patient safety, and that nurses are critical to quality care and the safety of patients. The importance of good working conditions and staffing for nursing services has been well established by research over the past decade.[33] The finding has been endorsed by the Institute of

Medicine,[34] a powerful opinion leader organization. The magnet status recognition movement, developed by the American Nurses Credentialing Center, has reinforced the connection between nursing services and hospital-patient outcomes. The Magnet Recognition Program® acknowledges healthcare organizations for nursing excellence as measured by quality patient care and innovations in professional practice. It is aimed at improving working conditions and the power and influence of nursing in hospitals.

Outcomes are improved when the right people are connected to the patient early in the disease process, and in many instances, nurse case managers are useful in making this happen. As nurses spend more time with patients than do physicians and other professionals, they are key "connectors" between what is actually happening with a patient and others who participate in their care. They are the hub of the interdisciplinary team. For example, in inpatient settings, the patient may tell the physician one thing, but the nurse may observe other, more subtle clues to the patient's condition. The nurse may then alert other health team members of the new information. In an era of heightened efforts to improve quality and safety, information exchange between professionals, departments and institutions is key, and nurses are central to communicating with and connecting to the right players.

A second trend that increases the value of nursing's connection to the patient is the series of innovations in service delivery meant to build services around the patient, rather than the provider. Service lines in hospitals, patient-centered care, family-centered care, and relationship-centered care all are variations on this enhanced patient focus. These developments, and the focus on the patient in nursing work, combine to make nursing a good background for organizational administration positions, enhancing nursing's input into organizational policy.[35] In many local settings, nurses, rather than physicians or administrators, have been the champions behind patient-centered care.[36]

Third, interprofessional or interdisciplinary, team-based care has become another major innovation in delivery settings and in the education of new healthcare practitioners. Again, nurses are ideally suited to facilitate such teams, because of their system orientation and the centrality of their role in the patient care system.

BOX 3: The Clinical Nurse Leader (CNL)

The CNL role is an innovative and controversial attempt by some individuals and groups in the nursing community to improve the lateral integration of patient care services (Begun, Tornabeni, & White, 2006). The CNL is called a lateral integrator because he or she follows the patient across a continuum of care, throughout the hospital setting. The CNL is a master's degree prepared nurse who assumes accountability for healthcare outcomes for a specific group of clients within a unit or setting through the assimilation and application of research-based information. The CNL serves as a lateral integrator for the healthcare team and facilitates, coordinates, and oversees the care provided by the healthcare team. The CNL is a "connector" role, centered on the patient. The role emerged under a variety of different titles and with some variation in many different workplaces in the 1990s, as healthcare organizations struggled to meet the challenge of improving patient quality and safety and controlling costs. In that way, the role emerged from the "shared sense-making" and "exploring" activities of working nurses and their colleagues from other communities of practice, particularly administration. Nurses themselves decided that this was an appropriate role for a nurse, and segments of the nursing community moved to implement it. ■

Nursing is using its connecting activities to explore new roles, like the CNL.[37] The CNL is the first new nursing role created since the 1980s, and it clearly is an interdisciplinary one, in which the nurse is responsible for coordinating diverse services for a group of patients. This recognizes nursing's ongoing connection to the patient, but adds a connection to the employing organization and a connection to interdependent professions. For additional reflections on the CNL movement, see Box 3.

Nurses serve a key connecting role in the care of chronically ill and dying patients. Lannamann et al. (forthcoming) suggest that providers stimulate conversations between patients, families and professionals to improve care for dying patients. Nurses often are employed as bereavement counselors, running support groups and facilitating linkages between patients and system resources. Nurses are in a perfect position to foster connections between patients, families, and other professionals to engage in such conversations.

Health informatics is an additional opportunity space for nursing in its connector role. Information systems that best serve holistic patient care need to be built around strong nursing input.

Conclusions: Nursing Leadership in the Larger Healthcare System

Drawing on its large size and scope, high demand, central locus in patient care, systems orientation, and a strong foundation of caring and earned trust, nursing is in the midst of an empowering transformation. The ascendance of nursing gives the profession a key position in shaping the healthcare system of tomorrow.

As the community of nursing enacts the competencies of complexity leadership, the reality of more potent influence in the larger healthcare community of practice emerges.

As the community of nursing enacts the competencies of complexity leadership, the reality of more potent influence in the larger healthcare community of practice emerges. The larger healthcare community consists of the practitioners, administrators, educators, suppliers, policymakers, and other stakeholders of the healthcare system, along with their organizations and associations. There is potential for new appreciation and acceptance of nursing as the health profession that contributes uniquely to the understanding of patients and their families and larger environments and thus should have valued input into shared sensemaking, exploring, and connecting activities of the larger healthcare delivery system.

Within organizations, this means that individual nurses are valued as partners who understand the organizational system in which they are embedded as well as the patient's system. This makes nurses ideal leaders of teams of professionals and collaboratives of patients and professionals. Nursing also provides a superb preparation for roles in organizational administration and in healthcare system policy-making. The same is true for the role of nursing organizations and associations—the nursing community's influence on reimbursement policy, health insurance policy, and other policies affecting patient care should be a more significant one.

It is a new era for the practice of nursing. Nursing is perfectly positioned to accomplish critical leadership tasks in a complex healthcare delivery system. A complexity-inspired approach to leadership recognizes that the future is unknowable and unpredictable, but that its emerging features are shaped by those individuals and organizations with the competencies to explore, connect, and make sense. Nurses and nursing organizations should embrace the opportunities to explore the future by taking risks and learning from them. Nurses and nursing organizations should embrace the opportunity to connect in new ways, not only to nursing colleagues and clients but also to administrators, policy-makers, other clinicians, and other stakeholders of the healthcare system. As they explore and connect, nurses and nursing organizations that choose to lead will be energized by making sense of the emerging world of nursing and healthcare in ways that fulfill the ideals of the profession of nursing.

> *A complexity-inspired approach to leadership recognizes that the future is unknowable and unpredictable, but that its emerging features are shaped by those individuals and organizations with the competencies to explore, connect, and make sense.*

Box 2: "The Most Modern Profession"

The following essay was written in 1991 and is reprinted from a weekly arts and entertainment newspaper based in Richmond, Virginia. It is an eloquently expressed appreciation of the nursing profession.

The Most Modern Profession
Dear Nurses,

I wish I were a nurse. I find it sad, not to be one. Millions of women like me have lived and grown older without joining your profession. What have we done with our lives? Too late: we made other choices. I am a retired hospital administrator, 60 years old and slowly, now, coming to terms with the fact that I will never be a nurse.

But I have a new privilege. I can observe the American way of health care from a distance, at least for now – long enough distance to put me at risk of being old-fashioned but also at an advantage, with a view of the whole greater than what one sees from a hospital office. And I am fortunate – lucky indeed – to be still close enough to the nursing profession to have a conversation.

Can we talk about the future of health care in America? Everyone else is talking about it. In fact, there's a lot more talk than action, but that is to be expected when big change is ahead and people begin to see that this is so.

America needs more nurses. Who else will rescue our floundering health care system?

On one level, it is obvious why we need more nurses. The current nurse shortage has left hospitals and nursing homes without enough nurses to take good comfortable time-generous care of patients, left home-care agencies and hospices scrounging for funds and begging nurses to join their special varied setting. But even if there were "enough" nurses we would still need more.

You have a way with information, a talent for complexity. I have watched a nurse talk an elderly hospital patient down from an agitated state during which he jerked his IV from his arm, wandered down the hall and pulled the fire alarm, then overturned the medication cart. She talked him down beyond the need for physical restraints. During their half-hour talk she got him through his daily corridor-walking exercise, put the IV back in, found out what was bothering him (a new pain had started in his abdomen that morning and he was afraid to mention it; his son had lost his job and his health insurance), rubbed his back, grabbed the doctor to examine him, called the local library for a video on support groups for the laid-off unemployed. This particular nurse holds a masters degree and a title: Clinical Specialist in Cardiac Care.

Specialists and generalists at the same time – how have you pulled this off? It is your talent for combining. Step by step, by asking questions – what does an isolation room really do to a psych patient? Why is a patient not taking his medicine? How much personal confidence and hope is needed to change one's eating habits? Putting pieces of information together, you have created a profession with a unique body of knowledge and skills without losing your traditional base of enthusiastic care. And with not much help from the rest of us.

Back in the old days when nursing was closer to the "handmaiden" image – when there were plenty of nurses who were expected to care for others simply because they were (mostly) women – you were, let's face it, not on everyone's mind. Dr. Lewis Thomas, a widely acclaimed writer of charming essays about medicine and science and himself, has called nurses "the glue that holds the hospitals together." The image lacks grace, it slaps you down at the corners, unable to move, stuck between other "visible" professions. Colorless, unseen, ubiquitous, inexpensive. Few of us think about glue until we need it so urgently we can do nothing further without it, then once used, it disappears from sight and mind. (I would have called you the central processing unit where information is received, understood, modified, augmented, timed, sent to the right station, brought back, put to bed, called up.)

Dr. Thomas means well. He knows that without you, hospitals could not function, things would fly apart if you were not holding on to them. But now you are no longer invisible. The serious shortage of nurses has put you out front. You literally had to disappear to be noticed.

Your newly acquired visibility calls for a new strategy.

Notice that front-page news articles on the cost and shortcomings of our health system are showing up thick and fast in national newspapers. The facts are familiar to you; you already know firsthand that our health-care system is full of cracks and holes. More than 33 million Americans have no health insurance. Catastrophe in the form of devastating illness is the financial ruin of many families. Long-term care for the elderly is marginal at best. Every year costs rise faster than inflation, and we now spend more than 12 percent of our gross national product on health care.

The system needs to be fixed, but not everyone agrees on how to do this. Do we adopt universal health coverage paid for by taxes, like that of Canada? Or should we patch up our current disorderly jumble of employer-based insurance and expand Medicaid for the poor? The issues will be access, cost and quality. Nurses have a track record for easing access, lowering cost and raising quality. How many times have you lightened an overwhelming fear of hospitals by sitting with a patient for an hour or more in the admitting office? How often have you chased down the one particular diagnostic test result that reduces the length of a hospital stay? Quality mixes it up, hospitals tell you when they are short of staff. How often have you – a cardiac nurse specialist – cross-covered in obstetrics, sat alone on the front line of a small hospital emergency room, then gone over to staff the long-term care unit where there are few emergencies, only the slow time-creep of chronic illness?

There is a large gap between current standards of quality and the true needs of the sick and elderly. Physicians and nurses have always known this and have always worked to close this gap. But today physicians are preoccupied. They see their Medicare fees reduced and their accountability increased. Change is harder on them than on you who are accustomed to deprivation.

In any new system, nurses will be called on to connect the loose ends, fill in the holes created by the rationing of high-cost technology. Some patients will have to wait for test, for surgery, for sophisticated treatment. These patients will need your knowledge – how long can one safely wait between a mastectomy and the start of chemotherapy? – your experience with pain control, your willingness to go out to their houses, your knack for sitting down in the middle of an anxious family that is bouncing off the walls and turning them into a group of reasonable adults.

Patients will need your quick informed access to the doctor – who, without admitting it, relies on you to keep on spinning your traditional protective web around clinical medicine.

Have nurses entered the debate on national health insurance? You have answers for us, your talents are required. I hope you are studying the proposals now in Congress, and I hope we will listen to what you have to say.

Take long-term care, for instance. Here in Virginia nurses travel to the far reaches of rural counties to seek out the frail elderly alone in their trailers – if loneliness were an airborne substance you would choke on it – and to shore up families trying to take care of their own with enormous sacrifices: jobs given up, privacy gone, money stretched. Your presence in their homes saves the health-care system millions of dollars: by expert advice, reassurance, encouraging informal networks for family and neighbors, respite, and friendship. Nursing homes thrive on your specialty in gerontology and your eclectic common sense.

A major change in our health-care system will bring its share of chaos, but this does not worry me as long as you are around turning chaos into order as you always have.

I won't go so far as to say that nothing matters except connection with our fellow human beings, but I can make a case for nursing as the most modern profession because of its connections. Ahead of its time, long into the future, beyond feminism, nursing is the model for the new technological society. The more information you have the more compassionate you become. What other profession can say that?

Wish I were one of you,

Susan Garrett

Susan Garrett lives in Charlottesville and writes about health care.
Reprinted with permission from Style Weekly, vol. 9, no. 26, June 25, 1991.

James W. Begun, PhD, is Hamilton Professor of Healthcare Management in the Division of Health Policy and Management, School of Public Health, University of Minnesota. A sociologist, Dr. Begun has written extensively on the evolution of health professions, including the book, *Strategic Adaptation in the Health Professions: Meeting the Challenges of Change.* Professor Begun is a member of the editorial boards of healthcare management journals, the Science Advisory Board of Plexus Institute, and Board of Directors of the Commission on the Accreditation of Healthcare Management Education.

Kenneth R. White, PhD, RN, FACHE, is Charles P. Cardwell, Jr. Professor of Health Administration, Director of the Graduate Program in Health Administration, and professor of nursing at Virginia Commonwealth University (VCU). Dr. White also holds faculty appointments at Luiss Business School in Rome, Italy and the Swiss School of Public Health, in Locarno, Switzerland. Dr. White has served on several hospital and health system boards. Dr. White is a registered nurse and a fellow and former governor of the American College of Healthcare Executives. He has published widely on hospital management and is co-author of *The Well-Managed Healthcare Organization.*

Works Cited

1. S. Kauffman, *At Home in the Universe: The Search for Laws of Self-Organization* (New York: Oxford University Press, 1995), 15.

2. W. H. Drath, "Leading Together: Complex Challenges Require a New Approach," in *The CCL Guide to Leadership in Action,* ed. M. Wilcox and S. Rush. (San Francisco: Jossey-Bass, 2004), 171-180, 177.

3. W. H. Drath, "The Third Way: A New Source of Leadership," in *The CCL Guide to Leadership in Action,* ed. S. Rush and M. Wilcox. (San Francisco: Jossey-Bass, 2004), 153-163.

4. W. H. Drath, *The Deep Blue Sea: Rethinking the Source of Leadership* (San Francisco: Jossey-Bass, 2001).

5. J. A. Raelin, *Creating Leaderful Organizations* (San Francisco: Barrett-Koehler, 2003).

6. J. Raelin, "Finding Meaning in the Organization," *MIT Sloan Management Review* 47, no. 3 (2006): 64-68.

7. J. P. Kotter, "Leading Change: Why Transformation Efforts Fail," *Harvard Business Review* 73, no. 2 (1995): 59-67.

8. E. E. Olson and others, *Facilitating Organization Change: Lessons from Complexity Science* (San Francisco: Jossey-Bass/Pfeiffer, 2001).

9. D. L. Cooperrider and D. Whitney, *Appreciative Inquiry: A Positive Revolution in Change* (San Francisco: Barrett-Hoehler, 2005).

10. Y. T. Shih, "Growth and Geographic Distribution of Selected Health Professions," *Journal of Allied Health* 29, no. 2 (1999): 61-70.

11. T. E. Sheets, *Encyclopedia of Associations* 35th ed., vol. 1 Part 2 (Farmington Hills: Gale Group, 1999).

12. P. I. Buerhaus, D. O Staiger, and D. I. Auerbach, "Implications of an Aging Registered Nurse Workforce," *JAMA* 283 (2000): 2948-2954.

13. E. O'Neil and J. Coffman, *Strategies for the Future of Nursing* (San Francisco: Jossey-Bass, 1998).

14. M. C. Mundinger et al., "Primary Care Outcomes in Patients Treated by NPs or Physicians," *JAMA* 283 (2000): 59-68.

15. Gallup Organization, "Nurses Top List of Most Honest and Ethical Professions," 2007. Available from www.galluppoll.com/content/?ci=25888&pg=1.

16. S. Reverby, "A Caring Dilemma: Womanhood and Nursing in Historical Perspective," *Nursing Research* 36 (1987): 5-11.

17. M. M. Leininger, *Care: The Essence of Nursing and Health* (Thorofare: Carles B. Slack, 1984).

18. J. Watson, *Nursing: The Philosophy and Science of Caring* (Boston: Little Brown, 1979).

19. J. Begun and K. White, "Altering Nursing's Dominant Logic: Guidelines From Complex Adaptive Systems Theory," *Complexity and Chaos in Nursing* 2, no. 5 (1995): 5-15, 6.

20. M. Snyder, E. C. Egan, and Y. Nojima, "Defining Nursing Interventions," *Image: Journal of Nursing Scholarship* 28 (1996): 137-141.

21. NANDA International, "History and Historical Highlights," Available from http://www.nanda.org/html/history2.html.

22. D. M. Doran, *Nursing-Sensitive Outcomes: State of Science* (Sudbury: Jones and Bartlett, 2003).

23. S. Nelson and S. Gordon, "Nurses Wanted: Sentimental Men and Women Need Not Apply," in *The Complexities of Care: Nursing Reconsidered* (Ithaca: Cornell University Press, 2006), 185-190, 190.

24. S. Jonas, *An Introduction to the U.S. Health Care System* 4th ed. (New York: Springer, 1998).

25. N. R. Barhydt-Wezenaar, "Nursing," in *Health Care Delivery in the United States*, ed. S. Jonas. 3rd ed. (New York: Springer, 1986), 90-124.

26. S. Ryan and S. Porter, "Men in Nursing: A Cautionary Comparative Critique," *Nursing Outlook* 41, no. 6 (1993): 262-267.

27. R. R. McDaniel and D. J. Driebe, "Complexity Science and Health Care Man-

agement," in *Advances in Health Care Management*, ed. J. D. Blair, M. D. Fottler, and G. T. Savage., vol. 2 (Stamford: JAI press, 2001), 11-36, 26.

28. J. S. Fulton and B. L. Lyon, "The Need for Some Sense Making: Doctor of Nursing Practice," 2007. Available from http://www.nursingworld.org/ojin/topic28/tpc28_3.htm.

29. B. R. Heller, M. T. Oros, and J. Durney-Crowley, "The Future of Nursing Education: Ten Trends to Watch," 2000. Available from www.nln.org/infotrends.

30. K. R. White, W. A. Wax, and A. Berry, "Accelerated Second Degree Advanced Practice Nurses: How Do They Fare in the Job Market?," *Nursing Outlook* 48 (2000): 218-222.

31. S. D. Roggenkamp and K. R. White, "For Nurse Entrepeneurs: What Motivated Them to Start Their Own Business," *Healthcare Management Review* 23, no. 3 (1998): 67-75.

32. K. R. White and J. W. Begun, "Nursing Entrepreneurship in an Era of Chaos and Complexity," *Nursing Administration Quarterly* 22, no. 2 (1998): 40-47.

33. L. H. Aiken et al., "Hospital Nurse Staffing and Patient Mortality, Nurse Burnout, and Job Dissatisfaction," *JAMA* 288, no. 16 (2002): 1987-1993.

34. Institute of Medicine, *Keeping Patients Safe: Transforming the Work Environment of Nurses* (Washington, D.C.: National Academies Press, 2004).

35. M. Arndt and B. Bigelow, "Hospital Administration in the Early 1990s: Visions for the Future and the Reality of Daily Practice," *Journal of Healthcare Management* 52, no. 1 (2007): 34-45.

36. S. Horowitz, "Creating Consensus: Partnering with Your Medical Staff," in *Putting Patients First: Designing and Practicing Patient-Centered Care*, ed. S. B. Frampton, L. Gilpin, and P. A. Charmel. (San Francisco: Jossey-Bass, 2003), 205-212.

37. J. W. Begun, J. Tornabeni, and K. R. White, "Opportunities for Improving Patient Care Through Lateral Integration: The Clinical Nurse Leader," *Journal of Healthcare Management* 51 (2006): 19-25.

38. K. E. Weick, *Sensemaking in Organizations* (Thousand Oaks: Sage, 1995)

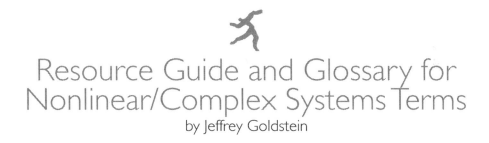

Resource Guide and Glossary for Nonlinear/Complex Systems Terms
by Jeffrey Goldstein

The development of the young science of complexity has been accompanied by an array of new concepts and terms. This section is designed to acquaint the reader with Complexity Science terms, many of which are used in the book. The description of each term in the Resource Guide and Glossary is accompanied by: first, a list of other relevant terms found in the glossary; and second, bibliographical references, with the complete list found at the end of the lexicon.

Adaptation:

In Darwin's Theory of Evolution, adaptation refers to the ongoing process by which an organism becomes "fit" to a changing environment. Adaptation occurs when modifications of an organism prove helpful to the survival of the species. These modifications result from both random mutations and recombinations of genetic material (for example, by sexual reproduction). Through the process of natural selection, the modifications that prove to aid in the survival of the organism may be selected for species survival as well. The idea of adaptation plays a very important role in the concept of a complex adaptive system, mostly associated with the Santa Fe Institute. Researchers at Santa Fe have suggested that natural selection operates on systems that already contain a great deal of emergent order. Adaptability is closely related to sustainability. Sustainable systems are ones that are capable of adaptation to a changing environment. The study of adaptation in various kinds of artificial life (see below) has demonstrated that adaptation may occur by some sort of change in the rules of interaction or the nature of interactions among the component agents. Thus, adaptation appears to consist in part of "learning" new rules through accumulating new experiences.

See: Complex, Adaptive Systems; Emergence; Genetic Algorithm
Bibliography: (Holland 1995); (Kauffman 1995); (Reid 2007).

Agent-based Models:

Computer simulations, derived largely from artificial life, which consist of semi-autonomous agents representing the factors being modeled and whose rules of interactions can be changed in order to see the emergent results. For example, the rules can be set up as either more cooperative or more competitive. The simulation is not expected to be a totally accurate representation of what is being modeled but, rather, to provide some insight into how changes in the rules can affect the outcomes observed. Agent-based models are becoming increasingly sophisticated, not only in terms of the possible range of agents' behaviors but also in terms of being embedded in richer environments that also play key roles in the ensuing simulation.

See: Artificial Life; Cellular Automata
Bibliography: (Axelrod 1984); (Axelrod & Cohen 2000); (Epstein 2007).

Artificial Life:

The life-like patterns emerging in cellular automata and related electronic arrays. These emergent patterns seem organic in the manner in which they move, grow, change their shape, reproduce themselves, aggregate, and die. Artificial life was pioneered by the computer scientist Chris Langton, and experimented with extensively at the Santa Fe Institute. Artificial life has been instrumental in the creation of agent-based models that are used to study various complex systems such as ecosystems, the economy, societies, cultures, and the immune system. The study of artificial life is promising insights into natural processes leading to the emergence of structure and new properties.

See: *Cellular Automata*
Bibliography: *(Langton 1986); For a new perspective (technical) on artificial life see (Griffeath and Moore, Eds. 2003).*

Attractor:

A mathematical construct very important to the field of nonlinear dynamical systems. Nonlinear or complex systems can be marked by a series of "phases," each of which displays the constraint of the behavior of the system in consonance with a reigning attractor(s). Such phases and their attractors can be likened (very loosely) to the stages of human development: infancy, childhood, adolescence, and so on. Each stage has its own characteristic set of behaviors, developmental tasks, cognitive patterns, emotional issues, and attitudes (although, of course, there is some variation among different people). Though a child may sometimes behave like an adult (and vice versa), the long term behavior is what falls under the sway of the attractor. Technically, in a dynamical system, an attractor is a pattern in phase or state space called a phase portrait that values of variables settle into after transient values die out as the system unfolds over time. More generally, an attractor can be considered a circumscribed or constrained range in a system that seemingly underlies and "attracts" how a system is functioning within particular environmental (internal and external) conditions. The dynamics of the system as well as current conditions determine the system's attractors. When attractors change, the behavior in the system changes because it is operating under a different set of governing principles. The change of attractors is called bifurcation, of which there are various kinds. A bifurcation results when there is a change in parameter values toward critical thresholds. Sometimes the latter criticalization is known as a far-from-equilibrium condition (particularly in the Prigogine School).

See: *Bifurcation, Far-from-equilibrium; Phase (State) Space*
Bibliography: *(Abraham 1982); (Goldstein 1994).*

Examples of Types of Attractors:
Fixed Point Attractor: An attractor that is a particular point in phase space, sometimes called an equilibrium point. As a point it represents a very limited range of possible behaviors in the system. For example, in a pendulum, the fixed point attractor represents the pendulum when the bob is at rest. This state of rest attracts the system because of gravity and friction. In an

organization a fixed point attractor would be a metaphor for describing when the organization is "stuck" in a narrow range of possible actions.

Periodic (Limit Cycle) Attractor: An attractor that consists of a periodic movement back and forth between two or more values. The periodic attractor represents more possibilities for system behavior than the fixed point attractor. An example of a period two attractor is the oscillating movement of a metronome. In an organization, a periodic attractor might be when the general activity level oscillates from one extreme to another. Or, an example from psychiatry might be bi-polar disorder where a person's mood shifts back and forth from elation to depression.

Strange Attractor: An attractor of a chaotic system is bound within a circumscribed region of phase space yet is aperiodic, meaning the exact behavior in the system never repeats. The structure of a strange attractor is fractal. A strange attractor can serve as a metaphor for creative activities in an organization in which innovation is possible yet there is a boundary to the activities determined by the core competencies of the organization as well as its resources and the environmental factors effecting the organization. A strange attractor portrays the characteristic of sensitive dependence on initial conditions (the butterfly effect) found in chaos.
    See: *Butterfly Effect; Chaos; Fractal; Sensitive Dependence on Initial Conditions.*
    Bibliography: *(Abraham 1982); (Ott 2003); For the slight technical difference between a strange and chaotic attractor see (Ott, Sauer, Yorke, 1994.)*

Basins of Attraction: If one imagines a complex system as a sink, then the attractor can be considered the drain at the bottom, and the basin of attraction is the sink's basin. Technically, it is the set of all points in phase space that are attracted to an attractor. More generally, the initial conditions of a system evolve into the range of behavior allowed by the attractor. When a specific attractor(s) is operative in a system, the behavior of the system will be consonant with that attractor(s), meaning that a measurement of that behavior will be in the system's basin of attraction and thereby eventually converge to the attractor(s), no matter how unusual the conditions affecting the system.

Autopoeisis:
A systems-based theory developed by the Chilean scientists Humberto Maturana and Francisco Varela. Maturana and Varela define a living organism as consisting of a circular, autocatalytic-like process which has its own survival as its main goal in a manner reminiscent of Kant's definition of causality in living systems versus that found in machines. An autopoeitic system's self-referential structure endows it with closure in the sense of being autonomous with respect to outside influences. The idea of closure

was developed to contrast with an overemphasis on openness in open systems theory. Autopoeisis is the main inspiration for the influential theory of social dynamics developed by Niklas Luhmann, which is more popular in Europe than in the USA. The management theorist Gareth Morgan points out that an organization's identity, strategies, and awareness of its market can be seen as an autopoeitic circularity. That is why organizations can get "stuck" in a rut of activity and become unadaptable to a changing environment.

See: Boundaries

Bibliography: (Chandler & Van de Vijver 2000); (Luhmann, Bednar, & Baecker 1996); (Maturana and Varela 1992); (Morgan 1997).

Benard System:

A simple physical system, consisting of a liquid in a container being heated from the bottom and which has been extensively studied by the Prigogine School because of it demonstration of self-organization and emergence. As the liquid in a container is heated from the bottom, at a critical temperature level (a far-from-equilibrium condition), there is the sudden emergence of striking hexagonally-shaped convection cells. Prigogine has termed these hexagonal cells "dissipative structures" since they maintain their structure while dissipating energy through the system and from the system to the environment. These "dissipative structures" are a good example of unpredictable emergent patterns since the direction of rotation of the convection cells is the result of the amplification of random currents in the liquid.

See: Dissipative Structures; Emergence; Far-from-equilibrium; Self-organization

Bibliography: (Nicolis 1989); (Nicolis and Prigogine 1989); (Goldstein 1994).

Bifurcation:

The emergence of a new attractor(s) in a dynamical, complex system that occurs when some parameter reaches a critical level (a far-from-equilibrium condition). For example, in the logistic equation or map system, bifurcation and the emergence of new attractors takes place when the parameter representing birth and death rates in a population reaches a critical value. More generally, a bifurcation is when a system shows an abrupt change in typical behavior or functioning that lasts over time. For example, a change of an organizational policy or practice which results in a long-term change of the business' or institution's behavior can be considered a bifurcation.

See: Attractor; Dynamical System; Far-from-equilibrium

Bibliography: (Abraham 1982); Guastello (1995).

Boundaries (Containers or "Closure"):

Processes of self-organization and emergence occur within bounded regions (e.g., the container holding the Benard System so that the liquid is intact as it undergoes far-from-equilibrium conditions). In cellular automata the container is the electronic network itself, which is "wrapped around" in that cells at the outskirts of the field are hooked back into the field. These boundaries or containers act to demarcate a system from its environment, and, thereby, maintain the identity of a system as it changes. Furthermore, boundaries channel the nonlinear processes at work during self-organization. In human systems, boundaries can refer to the actual physical plant, organizational policies, rules of interaction, and whatever serves to underlie an organization's identity and distinguish an organization from its environment. Boundaries need to be both permeable in the sense that they allow exchange between a system and its environments as well as impermeable in so far as they circumscribe the identity of a system in contrast with its environments.

See: Autopoeisis
Bibliography: (Chandler & Van de Vijver 2000); (Eoyang & Olson 2001); (Goldstein 1994); (Luhman, Bednarz, & Baecker 1996).

Butterfly Effect:

A popular image coming out of chaos theory which portrays the concept of sensitive dependence on initial conditions (i.e., a small change having a huge impact like a butterfly flapping its wings in South America which eventually leads to a thunderstorm in North America). Some attribute the term "butterfly" in "butterfly effect" to the butterfly-like shape of the phase portrait of the strange attractor discovered by the meteorologist Edward Lorenz when he first discerned what was later termed "chaos." The butterfly effect introduces a great amount of unpredictability into a system because one can never have perfect accuracy in determining those present conditions which will be amplified and lead to an outcome drastically different from the outcome expected. However, since chaotic attractors are not deterministic and not truly random and operate within a circumscribed region of phase or state space, there still exists a certain amount of predictability associated with chaotic systems. Thus, a particular state of the weather may be unpredictable more than a few days in advance; nevertheless, climate and season reduce the range of possible states of the weather, thereby adding some degree of predictability even into chaotic systems.

See: Chaos; Sensitive Dependence on Initial Conditions
Bibliography: (Abraham 1982); (Lorenz 1993); (Ott 2003).

Catastrophe Theory:

A mathematical theory of discontinuous change in a system formulated by the French mathematician René Thom from his work in algebraic topology. A "catastrophe" is an abrupt change in a variable(s) during the evolution of a system that can be modeled by structural equations and topological folds. Catastrophes are governed by control parameters whose change of values leads either to smooth transition at low values or abrupt changes at higher, critical values. For example, the way a dog's mood can change abruptly from playful to aggressive can be modeled by a simple "catastrophe." In organizations, the presence of sudden change can similarly be modeled using catastrophe theory. In recent years, catastrophe theory has come to be understood as a part of nonlinear dynamical systems theory.

See: Bifurcation
Bibliography: (Guastello 1995).

Cellular Automata:

One of the earliest species of artificial life, cellular automata are computer programs composed of a grid of "cells" (like a checkerboard), each cell of which turns on or off according to rules having to do with the on or off status of neighboring cells. For example, the rule might state that a cell be "on" if its four neighbor cells (east, west, north, and south) are also on. Emergent global patterns can then be observed that may move around the screen in a life-like manner (hence, "artificial life"). These emergent patterns can be quite complex although they emerge from very simple rules governing the connections among the cells. Early versions of cellular automata were conceived at the Institute for Advanced Study, Princeton, by eminent mathematicians as John von Neumann and Enrico Bomberi. The more familiar version was invented by the brilliant mathematician John Conway in his "Game of Life." Today, the study of cellular automata goes under the name artificial life (A-Life) because the exploration of cellular automata and their patterns at such places as the Santa Fe Institute has led to insights into the way structure is built-up in biological and other complex systems. Businesses and institutions can be modeled by cellular automata to the extent they are made up of interaction among people, equipment, and supplies. For example, the strength, number, and quality of connections among people or groups can be modeled by cells and rules among cells, so that how changes in the rules influence the emergence of patterns can be investigated. The hope is that cellular automata models will yield important insight into the dynamics of human systems.

See: Complexity; Emergence; Self-organization
Bibliography: (Dyson 1998); (Griffeath & Moore 2003); (Langton 1986); (Poundstone 1985).

Chaos:

A type of system behavior which although it displays random-like dynamics is actually deterministic, that is, underneath the apparent randomness is a hidden order or pattern. Chaos can be found in certain nonlinear dynamical systems when control parameters surpass certain critical levels. An often used example which has become something of an emblem for nonlinear dynamical systems is a nonlinear equation frequently used in populations studies. Changes in the key parameter value can result in a period-doubling route to chaos. The emergence of this kind of technically chaotic dynamic in a system suggests that simple rules can lead to complex results. Such systems are constituted by nonlinear, interactive, feedback relationships among the variables, components, or processes in the system. Chaotic time series of data from measurements of a system can be reconstructed or graphed in phase or state space as a chaotic or strange attractor with a fractal structure. Chaotic attractors are characterized by sensitive dependence on initial conditions so that although the behavior is constrained within a range, the future behavior of the system is largely unpredictable. However, unlike a random system which is also unpredictable, chaos is brought about by deterministic rules.

There is some measure of predictability due to the way the attractor of the system is constrained to a particular region of phase space. For example, if the weather is a chaotic system, particular states of the weather are unpredictable yet the range of those states is predictable. Thus, it is impossible to predict what the weather will be exactly on a particular date in August in New York, yet it is predictable that the temperature will fall within a range of 65-95 degrees Fahrenheit. That is, the climate acts as a constraint of the unpredictability of the state of the weather. In simulations of organizations, chaos has been seen to show up under certain circumstances, such as inventory or production processes, hospital admission rates, timing of procedures, and so on. Recent research has pointed to ways to control chaos by introducing particular perturbations into a system.

See: Attractor; Butterfly Effect; Control Parameter; Sensitive Dependence on Initial Conditions; Time Series

Bibliography: (Lorenz 1993); (Guastello 1995); (Ott 2003); (West 1990); (West 2006).

Chunking:

A term coined by journalist Kevin Kelly (past editor of *Wired* magazine) to describe how nature constructs complex systems from the bottom up with building blocks (systems) that have proven themselves able to work on their own. This concept is widely appreciated by evolutionary biologists and has been highlighted by complexity pioneer John Holland as a key feature of complex adaptive systems. Holland used the image of children's building blocks, of different shapes and sizes, combined in a variety of ways to yield new creations like castles and palaces.

See: Emergence; Genetic Algorithm; Self-organization
Bibliography: (Holland 1994); (Kelly 1994).

Co-evolution:

The coordinated and interdependent evolution of two or more systems within a larger system, such as different species co-evolving within a wider ecosystem. There is feedback among the systems in terms of competition or cooperation and different use of the same limited resources. An example of co-evolution may be how alterations in a predator can alter the adaptive possibilities of the prey. Co-evolution and co-creation are also found in social systems(e.g., businesses or institutions can co-evolve in various ways with their suppliers, receivers, even competitors in terms of joint ventures and strategic alliances).

Co-evolution is also seen in the theory of symbiogenesis described below in which two early life forms existing in an apparently host-parasite relationship merged to become the one cell prototype of all "modern" cellular structures.

See: Feedback; Fitness Landscapes
Bibliography: (De Duve, C. 2005); (Kauffman 1995); (Margulis & Sagan 2002); (Reid 2007).

Coherence:

The cohesiveness, coordination, and correlation characterizing emergent structures in self-organizing systems. For example, laser light is coherent compared to the light emanating from a regular light bulb. That emergent structures show a kind of order not found on the lower level of components suggests that complex systems contain potentials of functioning that have not been recognized before. Businesses and institutions can facilitate and utilize the coherence of emergent structures in place of the imposed kind of order found in the traditional bureaucratic hierarchy.

See: Dissipative Structures; Emergence; Self-organization; Synchronization
Bibliography: (Goldstein 1994); (Haken 1981); (Kauffman 1995); (Nicolis & Prigogine 1989); (Strogatz 2003).

Complexity:

A description of the complex phenomena demonstrated in systems characterized by nonlinear interactive components, emergent phenomena, continuous and discontinuous change, and unpredictable outcomes. Although there is at present no one accepted definition of complexity, the term can be applied across a range of different yet related system behaviors such as chaos, self-organized criticality, complex adaptive systems, neural nets, nonlinear dynamics, far-from-equilibrium conditions, and so on. Complexity characterizes complex systems as opposed to simple, linear, and equilibrium-based systems. There are many measures of complexity each differing according to the selected salient features of the system under investigation. Over the past two decades the sciences of complexity are increasingly being used to understand social system dynamics, including leadership, and human physiology.

See: *Complex, Adaptive Systems; Nonlinear System; Self-organization; Swarmware and Clockware*

Bibliography: *(Hazy, Goldstein, & Lichtenstein 2007); (Holland 1994); (Kauffman 1995); (Kelly 1994); (West 1990); (West 2006)*

Complex Adaptive System:

A complex, nonlinear, interactive system which has the ability to adapt to a changing environment. Such systems are characterized by the potential for the emergence of new structure with new properties. Complex adaptive systems (CASs) can evolve by random mutation, self-organization, the transformation of their internal models of the environment, and natural selection. Examples include living organisms, the nervous system, the immune system, the economy, corporations, societies, and so on. In a CAS, semi-autonomous agents interact according to certain rules, evolving to maximize some measure like fitness to their environment. The agents are diverse in both form and capability and they adapt by changing their rules and, hence, behavior, as they gain experience. Complex adaptive systems evolve historically, meaning they absorb their past history and experience, so that it affects their future trajectory. Their adaptability can either be increased or decreased by the rules shaping their interaction. Moreover, unanticipated, emergent structures can play a determining role in the evolution of such systems, which is why such systems show a great deal of unpredictability. A CAS has the potential for a great deal of creativity that was not programmed into them from the beginning. Considering an organization as a CAS shifts the way change is understood and approached. For example, change can be understood as the emergence of innovative structures resulting from enhanced interconnectivity as well as connectivity to the environment, the cultivation of diversity of viewpoint of organizational members, and the experimentation with alternative rules and structures.

See: *Agent-based Models; Adaptation; Emergence; Genetic Algorithm; Self-organization*

Bibliography: *(Holland 1994); (Kauffman 1995)*

Complex Responsive Processes

A way of understanding complex systems proposed by the organizational theorist Ralph Stacey to replace the technical and anti-humanistic bias he has argued underlies most studies of complex systems when applied to human dynamics. Building on the work of early social thinkers such as Norbert Elias and George Herbert Mead, as well as later psychodynamic theories, complex responsive processes have to do with how individual identity, behavior, and attitudes arise out of interactional dynamics in groups. Human interactions for Stacey are fundamentally comprised of symbolic communications, which encapsulate attitudinal dispositions of the body, behavior, emotions, and the mind. Rather than the complexity of human interaction being viewed through the lens of mechanical-style feedback, mathematical frameworks, or computational analogies, Stacey zeros in on the complexity of the communication webs linking people through their interactions. Out of interactions among persons arise social patterns that are sustained as well as changed by these interactions. From this perspective Stacey has reframed many complexity theory concepts as they relate to human behavior and interactions. One of the radical challenges he mounts involves questioning the existence of systems in human organizations of all types. In place of systems he contends are patterns of interactions that are maintained and changed through responsive processes among people in everyday relating.

See: Complex Adaptive Systems
Bibliography: (Mead 2002); (Stacey 2001); (Stacey 2007).

Deterministic System:

A system in which the later states of the system follow from or are determined by the earlier ones. Such a system is described in contrast to stochastic or random systems in which future states are not determined from previous ones. An example of a stochastic system would be the sequence of heads or tails of an unbiased coin or radioactive decay. If a system is deterministic, this doesn't necessarily entail that later states of the system are predictable from knowledge of the earlier ones. In this way, chaos is similar to a random system. For example, chaos has been termed "deterministic chaos" because, although it is determined by simple rules, its property of sensitive dependence on initial conditions makes a chaotic system largely unpredictable.

See: Chaos
Bibliography: (Lorenz 1993)

Difference/Diversity

Research has demonstrated that complex systems thrive on heterogeneity of their components or agents in relation to one another. For example, Steve Page has shown how differences or diversity of perspectives, stemming from such factors as ethnicity, background experience, academic training, can lead to more creative outcomes of working groups. In a similar vein, research in nursing homes by Ruth Anderson and colleagues suggest

that greater attention to interaction among different professionals—nursing assistants, RNs and nursing managers—and their different cognitive schema improve outcomes for patients.
   Bibliography: (Anderson, Issel, & McDaniel 2003); (Page 2007)

Difference Questioning: A group process technique developed by Jeffrey Goldstein that facilitates self-organization by generating far-from-equilibrium conditions in a work group. The process consists of several methods whereby information is amplified by highlighting the differences in perception, idea, opinion, and attitude among group members. Difference questioning does not aim at increasing or generating conflict, but, instead, tries to uncover the already differing standpoints. Moreover, the process takes place within boundaries that ensure the self-organization is channeled in constructive directions. Difference questioning aims at interrupting the tendency toward social conformity that robs groups of their creative idea generating and decision making potential. In other words, it strives to allow a greater flow of information among the group members which has been shown to be correlated with a far-from-equilibrium condition, a condition in which the emergence of new order can take place.
   See: Information; Self-organization
   Bibliography: (Goldstein 1994).

Dissipative Structure:
The term used by the Prigogine School (from Ilya Prigogine, winner of the Nobel Prize in chemistry) for emergent structures arising in self-organizing systems. Such structures are dissipative by serving to dissipate energy in the system. They happen at a critical threshold of far-from-equilibrium conditions. An example is the hexagonal convection cells that emerge in the Benard System when liquid in a container is heated. Other examples are the so-called "chemical clocks" demonstrated in the Belousov-Zhabotinsky reaction. These "chemical clocks" are composed of both temporal structures, such as a shift from one color to another, as well as spatial structures such as spiral waves. Hermann Haken, who founded the Haken School of Synergetics, uses the term "partly ordered", to describe phenomena similar to Prigogine's dissipative structure.
   The phrase "dissipative structure" cleverly juxtaposes two terms usually kept apart in thermodynamics circles: "dissipative" and "structure". "Dissipative" customarily refers to the loss of energy taking place during the transmutation of one kind of energy to another, for example, second law of thermodynamics and its central idea of entropy increase. Since an increase of entropy was eventually understood as a disintegrating tendency, "dissipative" then should carry connotations diametrically opposite to those of the building-up of "structure", since the latter denotes some kind

of endurance over time. Indeed, dissipative structures are often described as steady states, thus connoting something that is in a dynamic, rather than static equilibrium, or to use an analogy, like a vortex where its shape or organization remains intact although water molecules are in constant flux within it. By bringing these contrary terms together, Prigogine was calling attention to how in a dissipative structure heat transfer is not correlated with the dissolution of order but is actually the source of new order! Incidentally, one of Haken's terms for dissipative structures is "partly structured" again referring to the impermanent quality of these structures due to a constant flux of energy and matter passing through them.

   See: Coherence; Emergence; Far-from-equilibrium; Synchronization
   Bibliography: (Haken 1981); (Nicolis 1989); (Nicolis & Prigogine 1989).

Dynamical System:

A complex, interactive system evolving over time through multiple modes of behaviors. Instead of conceiving entities or events as static occurrences, the perspective of a dynamical system is of a changing, evolving process following certain rules and exhibiting an increase of complexity. This evolution can show transformations of behavior as new attractors emerge. The changes in a system's organization and behavior are called bifurcations. Dynamical systems are deterministic systems, although they can be influenced by random events. Times series data of dynamical systems can be graphed as phase portraits in phase space in order to indicate the "qualitative" or topological properties of the system and its attractor(s). For example, various physiological systems can be conceptualized as dynamical systems, the heart for one. Seeing physiological systems as dynamical systems opens up the possibilities of studying various attractor regimes. Moreover, certain diseases can be understood now as "dynamical diseases" meaning that their temporal phasing can be a key to understanding pathological conditions.

   See: Attractors; Bifurcation
   Bibliography: (Abraham 1982); (Guastello 1995)

Emergence:

The arising of new, unexpected structures, patterns, or processes in a self-organizing system. These emergents can be understood as existing on a higher level than the lower level components from which the emergents emerged. Emergents seem to have a life of their own with their own rules, laws, and possibilities unlike the lower level components. The term was first used by the nineteenth century philosopher G.H. Lewes and came into greater currency in the scientific and philosophical movement known as emergent evolutionism in the 1920's and 1930's. In an important respect the work connected with the Santa Fe Institute and similar facilities represents a more powerful way of investigating emergent phenomena. In organizations, emergent phenomena are happening ubiquitously yet their significance can be downplayed by control mechanisms grounded in the officially sanctioned corporate hierarchy. One of the keys for leaders from complex systems theory is how to facilitate emergent structures and take advantage of the ones that occur spontaneously.

Recently, such phenomena as disease, health and remission are being discussed as emergent phenomena in the sense that they arise out of "lower" level substrate conditions but express properties different than those found on the "lower" level.

See: Self-organization

Bibliography: (Cohen and Stewart 1994); (Goldstein 1999); (Goldstein 2006); Journal - Emergence: Complexity and Organization; (Goldstein 2007); (Richardson & Goldstein 2007).

Bibliography: Emergence in Biology – (Carroll 2005); (De Duve 2005); (Margulis and Sagan 2002); (Reid 2007); (Sole & Goodwin 2000;) Emergence in Physics – (Anderson 1972); (Laughlin 2006)

Equilibrium:

Equilibrium is a term indicating a rest state of a system, for example, when a dynamical system is under the sway of a fixed or periodic attractor. The concept originated in Ancient Greece when the great mathematician Archimedes experimented with levers in balance, literally "equilibrium". The idea was elaborated upon through the Middle Ages, the Renaissance and the birth of modern mathematics and physics in the seventeenth and eighteenth centuries. "Equilibrium" has come to mean pretty much the same thing as stability, i.e., a system that is largely unaffected by internal or external changes since it easily returns to its original condition after being perturbed, e.g., a balanced lever on a fulcrum (i.e., a see-saw). More generally, equilibrium suggests a system that tends to remain at status quo. The notion of physiological homeostasis, which has had such a strong hold in medicine and nursing could be considered a type of equilibrium.

See: Attractor; Far-from-equilibrium

Bibliography: (Goldstein 1994); (Nicolis & Prigogine 1989). (West 2006); Also, West's chapter in the current volume.

Far-from-equilibrium:

The term used by the Prigogine School for those conditions leading to self-organization and the emergence of dissipative structures. Far-from-equilibrium conditions move the system away from its equilibrium state, activating the nonlinearity inherent in the system. Far-from-equilibrium conditions are another way of talking about a criticalization in the values of parameters leading-up to a bifurcation and the emergence of new attractor(s) in a dynamical system.

See: Difference Questioning; Equilibrium; Self-organization
Bibliography: (Goldstein 1994); (Nicolis 1989).

Feedback:

The mutually reciprocal effect of one system or subsystem on another. Negative feedback is when two subsystems act to dampen the output of the other. For example, the relation of predators and prey can be described by a negative feedback loop because the growing number of predators leads to a decline in the prey population, but when prey decrease too much so does the population of predators because they will not have enough food. Positive feedback means that two subsystems are amplifying each other's outputs, such as the screech heard in a public address system when the microphone is too close to the speaker. The microphone amplifies the sound from the speaker which in turn amplifies the signal from the microphone and around and around. Feedback is a way of talking about the non-linear interaction among the elements or components in a system and can be modeled by nonlinear differential or difference equations as well as by the activity of cells in a cellular automata array. The idea of feedback forms the basis of system dynamics, a way of diagramming the flow of work in an organization founded by Jay Forrester and made popular by Peter Senge.

See: Interaction, Nonlinear
Bibliography: (Eoyang & Olson 2001)

Fitness Landscape:

The idea of epigenetic landscapes was proposed in the 1930's by the population geneticist Sewall Wright and then reformulated by others including the British biologist and embryologist C. H. Waddington. Wright, building on R. A. Fisher's notion that natural selection was the opposite of entropic dissipation, suggested a visual analogue to how selection worked genetically: genes were depicted in genotype "space" with organisms tied together into populations in an ecological "space." In such a landscape, there was not just one adaptive "peak" which genes had to "climb" in their adaptive strategies but rather a variety of them. An epigenetic landscape therefore combined into one image the themes of selection, population structure, and adaptation.

To portray how embryos would have a variety of possible pathways for development, Waddington imagined a similar landscape in which development took place, a landscape replete with contours like "hills" and "valleys" to represent channels carved-out by selectional pressures (in Waddington's terminology, "channeled" was referred to by "canalyzed"). The term "fitness landscape" was later adopted by Stuart Kauffman as a "graphical" way to measure and explore the adaptive (fitness) value of different configurations of some elements in a system. Each configuration and its neighbor configurations (i.e., slight modifications of it) are graphed as lower or higher peaks on a landscape-like surface (i.e., high fitness is portrayed as mountainous-like peaks, and low fitness is depicted as lower peaks or valleys). Such a display provides an indication of the degree to which various combinations add or detract from the system's survivability or sustainability. An important implication from studying fitness landscapes is that there may be many local peaks or "okay" solutions instead of one, perfect, optimal solution. The use of fitness landscapes can be applied to gain insight into various organizational issues including which innovative organizational designs, processes, or strategies promise greater potential.

See: Adaptation
Bibliography: (Weber & Depew 1994); (Kauffman 1995).

Fractal:

A geometrical pattern, structure, or set of points that are self-similar (exhibiting an identical or similar pattern) on different scales. For example, Benoit Mandelbrot, the discoverer of fractal geometry, describes the coast of England as a fractal, because as it is observed from closer and closer points of view (i.e., changing the scale), it keeps showing a self-similar kind of irregularity. Another example is the structure of a tree with its self-similarity of branching patterns on different scales of observation, or the structure of the lungs in which self-similar branching provides a greater area for oxygen to be absorbed into the blood. Strange attractors in chaos theory have a fractal structure. The imagery of fractals has been popularized by the fascinating graphical representations of fractals in the form of Mandelbrot and Julia Sets. Unlike the whole numbers characteristic of our usual dimensions (e.g., two or three dimensional drawings), the dimension of a fractal is not a whole number but a fractional part of a whole number such as a dimensionality of 2.4678.

Many measures of healthy physiologic complexity appear to show a fractal or fractal-like pattern in the sense of a similar or affine structure at different scales of resolution, for example: heart rate, breathing rate, blood counts. Degradation of the complexity of such patterns are also now thought to be associated with aging and many diseases and conditions, like Parkinson's disease, atrial fibrillation, congestive heart failure and cancer.

See also: Chaos
Bibliography: (Field & Golubitsky 1996); (Goldberger 1996); (Mandelbrot 1977); (Mandelbrot 1982); (Schroeder 1991); (West 1990); (West 2006).

Genetic Algorithm:

A type of evolving computer program developed by the computer scientist John Holland whose strategy of arriving at solutions is based on principles taken from genetics. Basically, the genetic algorithm uses the mixing of genetic information in sexual reproduction, random mutations, and natural selection at arriving at solutions. In an analogous manner to the way a genetic algorithm learns better solutions through the mixing of patterns and an openness to random or chance events, a complex, adaptive system can adapt to a changing environment through a mixing of previous internal models of their environment. Thus, genetic algorithms can provide insight into the creative process of problem solving or decision making.

See: Complex, Adaptive System; Randomness
Bibliography: (Eoyang & Olson 2001); (Holland 1994).

Graph Theory (Social Networks):

The mathematical theory that studies the properties of networks or webs of connections. A graph consists of edges (linkages) connecting nodes (what's connected). Examples of networks studied by graph theory include the internet, the economy, and genetic landscapes. Although graph theory is a purely mathematical discipline, the term is being included here because it is providing a theoretical foundation for the very influential and growing field of social network theory. The latter is providing rich insights into the dynamics of complex systems in general. For example, social network theory using graph theory has been discovering the complex structures of the internet, communities, employees connected within and outside their work organizations and so forth.

See: Scale-free Network; Small World Network
Bibliography: (Kilduff & Tsai 2003); (Newman, Barabasi, Watts 2006); (Trudeau 1993); (Watts 1999).

Information:

Originally, information in the technical senses referred to the bits of a message, as opposed to "noise," in a communication channel (formulated in Information Theory by the mathematician Claude Shannon building on earlier work done by Harry Nyquist and Ralph Hartley). Information has come to mean the bits of data that are the elements that are processed by the computer as information processor. "Noise" has a disorganizing effect in its way of disrupting redundant patterns so that novelty can come about in the emergent structures resulting from self-organizing processes. In terms of organizations, information is the cognate in social systems of what energy is in a physical system. According to Gregory Bateson, information is "a difference that makes a difference." In terms of social systems this refers to the differences among group members' perspectives on what is going on in the system. Information is not mere data: it is data that is meaningful to organizational members. An organization that is low in the flow of information is one in equilibrium or tending to maintain its status quo; whereas, an organization that is high in informational flow is in a far-from-equilibrium state in which dramatic changes can take place. Recent years have seen the birth of a new field entitled quantum information science which is playing an important role in the development of quantum computers and so-called quantum teleportation, both relying on the strange nature of quantum entanglement. These new fields reveal that information is increasingly seen as a basic constituent of the world around us or as the renowned physicist John Wheeler once put it, "It comes from bit!"

See: Redundancy
Bibliography: (Goldstein 1994); (Darling 2005).

Initial Conditions:

The state of a system corresponding to the beginning of a period of observing or measuring it. The initial conditions are what is assessed at any particular time, and to which one can compare any later observation, measurement, or assessment of the system as it evolves over time. For example, chaotic systems demonstrate sensitive dependence on initial conditions, meaning that the nonlinearity strongly amplifies slight differences in initial conditions, thereby rendering impossible the predictability of later states of the system.

See: Chaos; Sensitive Dependence on Initial Conditions
Bibliography: (Lorenz 1993); (Ott 2003).

Instability:

The condition of a system when it is more easily disturbed by internal or external forces or events, in contrast to a stable system that will return to its previous condition when disturbed. A pencil resting vertically on its eraser or a coin resting on its edge are examples of systems that have the property of instability because they easily fall over at the slightest breeze or movement of the surface they are resting on. An unstable system is one whose attractors can change, thus, instability is a characteristic of a system near or at bifurcation (or far-from-equilibrium).

See: Bifurcation; Equilibrium: Far-from-equilibrium
Bibliography: (Nicolis 1989)

Interaction:

The mutual effect of components or subsystems or systems on each other. This interaction can be thought of as feedback between the components as there is a reciprocal influence. In contrast, the effect of a pool cue on a cue ball is not interactive since the cue balls movement does not immediately affect the pool cue itself. For example, in cellular automata, it is the programmed rules that shape the kind of interaction occurring among neighboring cells. Complex adaptive systems are nonlinear, interactive systems.

See: Feedback; Nonlinear

Bibliography: (Eoyang and Olson 2001).

Linear System:

Technically, any system in which the change of values of its variables can be represented as a series of points suggesting a straight line on a coordinate plane, hence, the term "linear" for line. More generally, a linear system is one in which small changes result in small effects, and large changes in large effects. In a linear system, the components are isolated and noninteractive. Real linear systems are rare in nature since living organisms and their components are not isolated and are made-up of rich interactions.

See: Nonlinear System
Bibliography: (Abraham 1982)

Minimum Specifications:

The management theorist Gareth Morgan's term for processes encouraging self-organization by avoiding an overly top-down, imposed design on an organization or work group. These processes can include such elements as mission statements, guiding principles, boundaries, creative challenges, and so on. The key is for leadership to provide the minimum specifications so a work group itself has creative space to accomplish its work. Minimum specifications are analogous to the simple rules governing cell interactions in studies of cellular automata.

See: Cellular Automata; N/K Model
Bibliography: (Morgan 1997); (Zimmerman, Lindberg, Plsek 2001).

Neural Networks:

Electronic automatons, similar in some ways to cellular automata, that offer a simplified model of a brain. As such, neural networks are devices of machine learning that are based on associative theories of human cognition. Using various algorithms and weightings of different connections between "neurons," they are set up to learn how to recognize a pattern such as learning a voice, recognizing a visual pattern, learning some form of robotic control, manipulating symbols, or making decisions, and so on. Generally, neural nets are composed of three layers: input neurons; output neurons; and a layer in-between where information from input to output is processed. Initially the network is loaded with a random program, then the output is measured against a desired output which prompts an adjustment in the "weights" assigned to the connectivities in response to the "error" between the actual and desired output, and this is repeated many times. In this way, the neural network learns. In a sense, a neural net has to be able to discover its own rules. Changing the rules of interaction between the "neurons" in the network can lead to interesting emergent behavior.

Hence, neural nets are another tool for investigating self-organization and emergence.

See: *Adaptation*
Bibliography: *(Allman 1989).*

Nonlinear System (Nonlinearity):

Technically, any system where the data points representing values of its variables can be represented as a curvilinear pattern on a coordinate plane, hence, "*nonlinear*" for not-a-line. That is, the system's dynamics are more appropriately represented by nonlinear and not linear functions. More generally, a system in which small changes can result in large effects, and large changes in small effects. Thus, sensitive dependence on initial conditions (the butterfly effect) in chaotic systems illustrates the extreme nonlinearity of these systems. In a nonlinear system the components are interactive, interdependent, and exhibit feedback effects. Complex adaptive systems are nonlinear systems.

Before the advent of chaos and complexity theories during the past thirty-five years, nonlinear functions were mostly relegated to appendices in textbook because of their refractoriness to analytic solutions. But now, because of both advances in computational approaches to nonlinear functions and the recognition of the crucial role played by interactions in most systems of interest, it is increasingly recognized that examples of nonlinear systems are presumably endless. Thus, human physiology is replete with nonlinear systems, such as the cardiac, circulatory, and immune systems. In addition, in social systems nonlinearity seems to be the norm since they are constituted by mutually reciprocal interactions among the members of social groupings and such interactions are appropriately modeled by nonlinear rather than linear equations.

See: *Linear; Sensitive Dependence on Initial Conditions*
Bibliography: *(Eoyang and Olson 2001); (Goldstein 1994); (Guastello 1995); (Scott 2005); (West 1990); (West 2006).*

Novelty:

One of the defining characteristics of emergent patterns is their novelty or innovative character. Indeed, that is why such phenomena are termed "emergent" since they introduce new qualities into the system that were not pre-existing in it. An example is the novel nature of the "dissipative structures" that arise in nonlinear systems at far-from-equilibrium conditions. This novelty is neither expected, predictable, nor deducible from the pre-existing components. Moreover, this novelty is not reducible to the lower level components without loosing its essential characteristics. An issue, therefore, for practitioners working with complex systems, is to determine which system processes are necessary for the emergence of novelty. That is, novel outcomes demand novel processes that prompt a system to produce novel structures and practices. In organizations, novel emergent outcomes are typically termed innovations. The study of the diffusion of innovations was pioneered by the late Everett Rogers (see below).

See: *Bifurcation; Emergence; Far-from-equilibrium; Self-organization*
Bibliography: *(Goldstein 2006); (Rogers 2003); (Van de Ven & Garud 1994).*

Parameters:

Variables in the mathematical equations used to model system behavior. Changes in the values of these variables can affect the system's behavior. *Control Parameters:* These parameters often model some kind of external influence on a system that facilitate a far-from-equilibrium condition or, in other words, expedite a bifurcation. An example is temperature in the Benard System, which at a critical value prompts self-organization and the emergence of hexagonal convection cells when a particular liquid in a container is heated from the bottom.

Order Parameters: Parameters that represent some global emergent characteristic of a system as opposed to variables of lower level components. The shift to order parameters signifies recognition that emergent phenomena need to be investigated on their own terms.

Lambda Parameter: A parameter used by the computer scientist Chris Langton to get at the range where self-organization is most likely in cellular automata. As such the lambda parameter is a control parameter.

See: *Bifurcation; Cellular Automata*
Bibliography: *(Haken 1981); (Langton 1986).*

Phase (State) Space:

An abstract mathematical space which is used to display time series data of the measurements of a system. The dimensions of phase or state space correspond to the number of variables used to characterize the state of the system. For example, the phase space of a pendulum would consist of two dimensions: the speed of the bob; and the distance of the bob from the vertical resting state. Phase space is very helpful for observing the patterns that result as systems evolve over time. Please note that time is usually not one of the explicit dimensions of the phase space, a role that time does play in a straight graphical depiction of a time series.

Phase Portrait: The geometrical patterns shown in phase space as a system evolves. These portraits may be attractors such as fixed point, periodic, and strange attractors. They can also include repellors (the opposite of attractors) and such interesting patterns as saddles (in which there are attractor(s) in one direction and repellor(s) in another direction) and separatrices, or boundaries between two basins of attraction.

See: Attractors; Chaos
Bibliography: (Yates, et. al. 1987); (Guastello 1995)

Positive Deviance:

Experiments or deviations from the norm in a social system that can lead to positive change. The phrase itself "positive deviance" is a kind of oxymoron, since it pairs the constructive term "positive" with the negative term "deviance," the latter term carrying quite a bit of pejorative associations precisely because it pertains to deviations from the norm. For example, members of a society practicing "fringe behavior" are often called deviants. However, branding "deviance" with such derogatory outcomes sets up a bias that protects the norm with a halo of righteousness while condemning deviations-from-the-norm as degenerate. If this bias were strictly enforced, we would never have gained most of the great scientific and social advances of human history. All such major innovations and transformations, in one way or another, relied on radical departures from the norm. Both the Copernican and the American Revolutions are cases in point.

A social interventional method termed "Positive Deviance" developed by Jerry and Monique Sternin identifies novel experiments in complex social systems—deviations from the norm—and harnesses them to generate positive outcomes. "Radical" ideas from organizational outliers are reframed as solutions with the potential of bringing about significant social system change. According to Jerry Sternin, in many communities facing seemingly intractable problems, there are certain individuals or groups (positive deviants) with the same access to resources as other community members whose special practices, strategies or behaviors generate better results.

Bibliography: (Sternin & Choo 2000); (Sternin 2003).

Power Laws:

A type of mathematical pattern in which the frequency of an occurrence of a given size is inversely proportionate to some power (or exponent) of its size. For example, in the case of avalanches or earth quakes, large ones are fairly rare, smaller ones are much more frequent, and between these extremes are cascades of different sizes and frequencies which take place a moderate number of times. Power laws define the distribution of catastrophic events in self-organized critical systems. Systems with power law distributions are marked by invariance with respect to scale and universality, the latter term referring to remarkably similar dynamics across quite different systems. Power laws are associated with fractal-like patterns since the pattern is self-similar with respect to scale. In this regard power law signatures have been discovered in heart inter-beat variability and are suspected in many other physiological phenomena.

See: Fractal; Scale-free Network; Self-organized Criticality; Sensitive Dependence on Initial Conditions

Bibliography: (Bak 1996); (Barabási 2002); (Schroeder 1991); (West 2006).

Redundancy:

The existence of repetitive patterns or structures. In an important sense, redundancy refers to order in a complex system in the sense that order is defined as the existence of structures that maintain themselves over time (i.e., they are stable). In information theory, redundancy refers to repetition in patterns of messages in a communication channel. If the message contains these redundancies, they can be compressed further. For example, if a message contains a series of two hundred and fifty 1s, then the message could be compressed into a command which effectively says "and then repeat 1 250 times" instead of writing out all two hundred fifty 1s. Self-organizing processes demand some element of redundancy which can be considered as a "fuel" for the processes leading to emergence. In other words, novel patterns come from a recombination of redundant patterns.

See: Information; Novelty

Bibliography: (Campbell 1982); (Poundstone 1985).

Scale:

The level at which a system is observed. For example, one can observe the coast of England from a satellite or from a jet liner or from a low flying plane, or from walking along the coast, or from peering down into the sand and rocks on a cove beach that you are standing on. Each of these perspectives is of a different scale of the actual coast of England. Fractals are geometric patterns that are self-similar on different scales.

See: Fractal; Power Law

Bibliography: (Kaye 1989); (Schroeder 1991)

Scale-free Network

A type of network, studied by means of graph theory, in which some of the nodes act as highly connected hubs but most other nodes have a lower degree of connectivity. They are called "scale-free" because their structure and dynamics are independent of the system's size defined in terms of number of nodes. A scale-free network has the same features no matter what number of nodes is in the network. Scale-free networks also exhibit a power law distribution and may be more resilient in the face of loss of connectednes than hub networks which cannot withstand the loss of the hub.

See: Fractal; Scale; Graph Theory; Small Worlds

Bibliography : (Barabási 2002); (Watts 1999).

Self-organization:

A process in a complex system whereby new emergent structures, patterns, and properties arise without being externally imposed on the system. Not controlled by a centralized, hierarchical "command and control" center, self-organization is usually distributed throughout a system. Self-organization requires a complex, nonlinear system under appropriate conditions, variously described as "far-from-equilibrium" or criticalization. Studied in physical systems by Ilya Prigogine and his followers, as well as the Synergetics School founded by Hermann Haken, self-organization is now studied primarily through computer simulations such as cellular automata, Boolean networks, and other phenomena of artificial life. Self-organization is recognized as a crucial way for understanding emergent, collective behavior in a large variety of systems including: the economy; the brain and nervous system; the immune system; ecosystems; and the modern large corporation or institution. The emergence of new system order via self-organization is thought to be a primary tendency of complex systems in contrast to the past emphasis on the degrading of order in association with the principle of entropy (second law of thermodynamics). In recent perspectives, rather than fighting against entropy, self-organization can be understood as a way that the total entropy of a complex system along with its environment(s) increases.

Now that we have a better handle scientifically on how self-organization takes place, it is easier to recognize instances of it in the world around us. For example, self-organization could be an appropriate way of understanding how a hospital staff may spontaneously re-organize itself to respond more effectively to a sudden influx of critically ill patients. This is what seems to have happened, for example, at Beekman Downtown Hospital in Manhattan during the tragedy of 9-11-2001 when the staff coalesced into novel treatment teams to handle the tremendous inflow of seriously wounded victims. Self-organization may also take place in innumerable other ways, for example, the change in family dynamics that results when a family member enters a hospice program, or the emergence of novel ways to provide care to a seriously ill that comes from interactions among the patient, nurses, physicians, other healthcare professionals, support staff and family members when patients have multiple chronic diseases.

See: Coherence; Dissipative Structures; Emergence; Far-from-equilibrium
Bibliography: (Eoyang & Olson 2001); (Goldstein 1994); (Nicolis 1989); (Nicolis & Prigogine 1989).

Self-organized Criticality:

Formulated by the late physicist Per Bak, a phenomenon of sudden change in physical systems in which they evolve naturally to a critical state at which abrupt changes can occur. That is, when these systems are not in a critical state (i.e., they are characterized by instability), output follows from input in a linear fashion, but when in the critical state, systems characterized by self-organized criticality act like nonlinear amplifiers, similar to but not as extreme as the exponential increase in chaos due to sensitive dependence on initial conditions. That is, the nonlinear amplification in a self-organized, critical system follows a power law instead of an exponential law. Such systems are self-organized in the sense that they reach a critical state on their own. Examples of such systems include avalanches, plate tectonics leading to earthquakes or stock market systems leading to crashes. Because these systems follow power laws, and because fractals also show a similar mathematical pattern, it may be that many naturally occurring fractals, such as tree growth, the structure of the lungs, and so on, may be generated by some form of self-organized criticality.

See: Bifurcation; Catastrophe; Instability; Power Law; Self-organization
Bibliography: (Bak 1996).

Sensitive Dependence on Initial Conditions:

The property of chaotic systems in which a small change in initial conditions can have a hugely disproportionate effect on outcome. Sensitive dependence on initial conditions is popularly captured by the image of the butterfly effect. Sensitive dependence on initial conditions makes the behavior of chaotic systems largely unpredictable because measurements at initial conditions always will contain some amount of error. The late mathematical metereologist Edward Lorenz uncovered this concept in his work on weather forecasting. He noticed that a seemingly insignificant difference in an initial parameter in a forecasting system modeled on his computer led to very different forecasts.

See: Chaos; The Butterfly Effect
Bibliography: (Lorenz 1993); (Ott 2003).

Small World Network:

A type of graph network in which the connectivity among nodes leads to the formation of pathways linking an unusually large number of nodes. The small world phenomenon was made famous in the play(movie) "Six Degrees of Separation" and the "Kevin Bacon number", which refers to the idea that any actor can be linked through his or her film roles to the actor Kevin Bacon. In both of these, it has been shown mathematically and through experimentation that nearly everyone on the planet is remarkably linked by no more than six linkages in a network comprising all the relationships between people.

See: Graph Theory; Scale-free Network
Bibliography: (Barabási, A. L. 2002); (Watts 1999).

Stability:

The opposite of "instability," the property of a system which stays pretty much the same after being disturbed by internal or external forces or events. For example, the deeper the keel of a sailboat, the more stable it is regarding the wind and currents. A running gyroscope is stable with respect to changes affecting its centrifugally determined level plane. Stability is sometimes used as a synonym for equilibrium or with the state of a system circumscribed within a particular attractor regime.

See: Equilibrium; Far-from-Equilibrium; Instability
Bibliography: (Nicolis 1989); (Nicolis & Prigogine 1989); (Ott 2003).

Swarmware and Clockware:

Two terms coined by the editor of Wired Magazine Kevin Kelly for two antithetical management processes. "Clockware" are rational, standardized, controlled, measured processes; whereas "swarmware" are processes including experimentation, trial and error, and risk-taking. Clockware processes are seen in linear systems whereas swarmware is what happens in complex systems undergoing self-organization as a result of the nonlinear interaction among components.

See: Cellular Automata; Complex Adaptive System; Self-organization
Bibliography: (Kelly 1994).

Symbiogenesis:

A theory about the emergence of new biological forms put forward by Lynn Margulis which posits that cooperation or symbiosis among two or more distinct types of organisms can lead to the emergence of radically novel types of organisms. It is believed that primitive organisms called eukaryotes incorporated certain elements of the aerobic bacteria that had been ingested into them and that out of this symbiotic relation, the more advanced prokaryotic cells resulted with the novel features of nuclei and membranes. Symbiogenesis manifests a new interpretation of evolution whereby other mechanisms besides variation and selection may be at work. It also represents a growing recognition of the importance of cooperative relationships among species instead of the more typical emphasis on competition and predator-prey relationships.

See: Co-evolution; Emergence
Bibliography: (De Duve 2005); (Margulis & Sagan 2002); (Reid 2007)

Synchronization:

A phenomenon that can occur in complex systems in which system components or agents align themselves in a startling coherence. A striking example can be seen in the dramatic synchronization of lighting in certain species of fireflies (what we used to call "lightning bugs" as children). This can be seen inside the Great Smoky National Park near Elmont, Tennessee, during mid-June at about 10 PM every night when thousands of fire flies flash together according to a highly synchronized pattern: After six seconds of total darkness, thousands of lights flash in perfect synchrony six times in three short seconds; the pattern then repeats itself over and over again. A similarly synchronization of firing among fireflies can be observed in parts of Thailand. Research has shown that synchronization takes place without any "leader" firefly. Instead synchronization develops out of the interaction among the fireflies. Specifically, under the right conditions, signals from one to the other become resonated in concert. In human systems, synchronization is evident during sporting events when fans in a stadium combine movement into the famous "wave" of hands.

A destructive kind of synchronization was responsible for the collapse of the Tacoma Narrows Bridge on December 11, 1940. A confluence of high winds and too much structural coherence that was built into the bridge led to a resonance of vibrations affecting the bridge leading to the collapse of the bridge's structure.

See: Coherence
Bibliography: (Strogatz 2003)

Time Series:
A collection of measurements of the variable(s) of a system as it evolves over time. Traditionally, times series data were graphed with time on the x-axis and some system variable on the y-axis. For example, the time series of an oscillating (periodic) system such as a forced pendulum or a metronome would show a curve depicting the speed of the pendulum bob going up and down like hills and valleys over time. However, as the result of dynamical systems theory, time series are now usually graphed in phase or state space with either two or more variables marking each dimension, or one variable is mapped against a time lagged version of the same variable. By graphing times series data in phase space, attractors can be identified more easily. Our ability to graph such times series and to determine their attractors has been greatly accelerated by the rise of the personal computer.

See: Attractor; Phase Space
Bibliography: (Guastello 1995); (Ott, Sauer, Yorke 1994)

Jeffrey Goldstein, PhD, is professor at the School of Business, Adelphi University. Dr. Goldstein specializes in the application of complexity theory to organizations. His book of 1994 on this subject, *The Unshackled Organization,* was hailed by Industry Week as a "fascinating vision." Professor Goldstein is co-editor-in-chief of *Emergence: Complexity & Organization,* the only journal currently devoted to the applications of the sciences of complex systems to organizations. He serves as a trustee of The Society for Chaos Theory in Psychology and the Life Sciences, as a member of the Science Advisory Board of Plexus Institute, and as a fellow of the Institute for the Study of Coherence and Emergence.

Works Cited

- *Encyclopedia of Nonlinear Science* (New York: Routledge, 2005).

- R. Abraham, *Dynamics: The Geometry of Behavior* (Santa Cruz: Aerial Press, 1982).

- W. F. Allman, *Apprentices of Wonder: Inside the Neural Network Revolution* (New York: Bantam Books, 1989).

- P. Anderson, "More Is Different: Broken Symmetry and the Nature of the Hierarchical Structure of Science," *Science* 177, no. 4047 (1972): 393-396.

- R. Anderson, L. Issel, and R. McDaniel, "Nursing Homes As Complex Adaptive Systems: Relationship Between Management Practice and Resident Outcomes," *Nursing Research* 52, no. 1 (2003): 12-21.

- R. Anderson, L. Issel, and R. McDaniel, "Relationship Between Management Practice and Resident Outcomes," *Nursing Research* 52, no. 1 (2003): 12-21.

- R. Axelrod, *The Evolution of Cooperation* (New York: Basic Books, 1984).

- R. Axelrod and M. Cohen, *Harnessing Complexity: Organizational Implications of a Scientific Frontier* (New York: Basic Books, 2000).

- P. Bak, *How Nature Works: The Science of Self-Organized Criticality* (New York: Springer-Verlag, 1996).

- A. L. Barabasi, *Linked: The New Science of Networks* (Cambridge: Perseus, 2002).

- J. Campbell, *Grammatical Man: Information Theory, Entropy, Languages, and Life* (New York: Simon Shuster, 1982).

- S. Carroll, *Endless Forms Most Beautiful: The New Science of Evo Devo* (New York: W. W. Norton & Co., 2005).

- J. Chandler and G. Van de Vijer, *Closure: Emergent Organizations and their Dynamics* (New York: The New York Academy of Sciences, 2000).

- D. Darling, *Teleportation: The Impossible Leap* (Hoboken: John Wiley and Sons, 2005).

- C. DeDuve, *Singularities: Landmarks on the Pathways of Life* (New York: Cambridge University Press, 2005).

- G. Dyson, *Darwin Among the Machines: The Evolution of Global Intelligence* (New York: Basic Books, 1998).

- G. Eoyang and E. Olson, *Facilitating Organizational Change: Lessons from Complexity Science* (San Francisco: Jossey-Bass/Pfeiffer, 2001).

- J. Epstein, *Generative Social Science: Studies in Agent-Based Computational Modeling*, Princeton Studies in Complexity (Princeton: Princeton University Press, 2007).

- M. Field and M. Golubitsky, *Symmetry in Chaos: A Search for Patterns in Mathematics, Art and Nature* (New York: Oxford University Press, 1996).

- A. Goldberger, "Nonlinear Dynamics for Clinicians: Chaos Theory, Fractals and Complexity at the Bedside," *The Lancet* 347 (1996): 1312-1314.

- J. Goldstein, *The Unshackled Organization* (Portland: Productivity Press, 1994).

- J. Goldstein, "Emergence As a Construct: History and Issues," *Emergence* 1, no. 1 (1999): 49-7278.

- J. Goldstein, "Emergence, Creative Process, and Self-Transcending Constructions," in *Managing Organizational Complexity: Philosophy, Theory, and Application*, ed. K. Richardson. (Greenwich: Information Age Press, 2006), 63-78.

- J. Goldstein, "A New Model for Emergence and its Leadership Implications," in *Complex Systems Leadership Theory: New Perspectives From Complexity Science on Social and Organizational Effectiveness*, ed. J Hazy, J. Goldstein, and B. Lichtenstein. (Mansfield: ISCE Publishing, 2007), 62-93.

- D. Griffeath and C. Moore, *New Constructions in Cellular Automata* (New York: Oxford University Press, 2003).

- S. Guastello, *Chaos, Catastrophe, and Human Affairs: Applications of Nonlinear Dynamics to Work, Organizations, and Social Evolution* (Mahwah: Lawrence Erlbaum Associates, 1995).

- S. Guastello, *Managing Emergent Phenomena: Nonlinear Dynamics in Work Organizations* (Mahwah: Lawrence Erlbaum Associates, 2001).

- H. Haken, *The Science of Structure: Synergetics* (New York: Van Nostrand Reinhold, 1981).

- J. Hazy, J. Goldstein, and B. Lichtenstein, *Complex Systems Leadership Theory: New Perspectives from Complexity Science on Social and Organizational Effectiveness* (Mansfield: ISCE Publishing, 2007).

- J. Holland, *Hidden Order: How Adaptation Builds Complexity* (Reading: Addison-Wesley, 1994).

- J. Holland, *Hidden Order: How Adaptation Builds Complexity* (Reading: Addison-Wesley, 1995).

- J. Holland, *Emergence: From Chaos to Order* (Reading: Addison-Wesley, 1998).

- S. Kauffman, *The Origins of Order: Self-Organization and Selection in Evolution* (New York: Oxford University Press, 1993).

- S. Kauffman, *At Home in the Universe: The Search for Laws of Self-Organization* (New York: Oxford University Press, 1995).

• B. H. Kaye, *A Random Walk Through Fractal Dimensions* (New York: VCH Publishers, 1989).

• K. Kelly, *Out of Control: The New Biology of Machines, Social Systems, and the Economic World* (Reading: Addison Wesley Longman, 1995).

• M. Kilduff and W. Tsai, *Social Networks and Organizations* (Thousand Oaks: Sage, 2003).

• C. G. Langton, "Studying Artificial Life with Cellular Automata," in *Evolution, Games, and Learning: Models for Adaptation in Machines and Nature*, ed. D. Farmer et al. (Amsterdam: North-Holland, 1986), 120-149.

• R. Laughlin, *A Different Universe: Reinventing Physics from the Bottom Down* (New York: Basic Books, 2006).

• E. Lorenz, *The Essence of Chaos* (London: UCL, 1993)

• N. Luhmann, J. Bednarz, and D. Baecker, *Social Systems* (Palo Alto: Stanford University Press, 1996).

• B. B. Mandelbrot, *Fractals, Form, Chance and Dimension* (San Francisco: W.H Freeman and Co., 1977).

• B. B. Mandelbrot, *The Fractal Geometry of Nature* (San Francisco: W.H. Freeman and Co., 1982).

• L. Margulis and D. Sagan, *Acquiring Genomes: A Theory of the Origins of Species* (New York: Basic Books, 2002).

• H. Maturana and F. Varela, *Autopoeisis and Cognition* (Boston: D. Reidel, 1980).

• H. Maturana and F. Varela, *The Tree of Knowledge: The Biological Roots of Human Understanding* (Boston: New Science Library, 1987).

• G. H. Mead, *The Philosophy of the Present* (Amherst: Prometheus Books, 2002).

• G. Morgan, *Images of Organization* (Thousand Oaks: Sage, 1997).

• M. Newman, A. Barabasi, and D. Watts, *The Structure and Dymanics of Networks* (Princeton: Princeton University Press, 2006).

• G. Nicolis and I. Prigogine, *Exploring Complexity: An Introduction* (New York: W.H. Freeman and Company, 1989).

• G. Nicolis, "Physics of Far-From-Equilibrium Systems," in *The New Physics*, ed. P. Davies. (Cambridge: Cambridge University Press, 1989).

• E. Ott, T. Sauer, and J. Yorke, *Coping with Chaos: Analysis of Chaotic Data and the Exploitation of Chaotic Systems* (Somerset: Wiley-Interscience, 1994).

• E. Ott, *Chaos in Dynamical Systems* (Cambridge: Cambridge University Press, 2003).

• S. Page, *The Difference: How the Power of Diversity Creates Better Groups* (Princeton: Princeton University Press, 2007).

* W. Poundstone, *The Recursive Universe: Cosmic Complexity and the Limits of Scientific Knowledge* (Chicago: Contemporary Books, 1985).

* R. Reid, *Biological Emergences: Evolution by Natural Experiment* (Cambridge: MIT Press, 2007).

* K. Richardson and J. Goldstein, *Classic Complexity: From the Abstract to the Concrete* (Mansfield: ISCE, 2007).

* E. Rogers, *Diffusion of Innovation* 5 ed. (New York: Free Press, 2003).

* M. Schroeder, *Fractals, Chaos, Power Laws: Minutes from an Infinite Paradise* (New York: W.H. Freeman & Co., 1991).

* R. Sole and B. Goodwin, *Signs of Life: How Complexity Pervades Biology* (New York: Basic Books, 2000).

* R. Stacey, *Complex Responsive Processes in Organizations: Learning and Knowledge Creation* (London: Routledge, 2001).

* R. Stacey, *Strategic Management and Organisational Dynamics: The Challenge of Complexity to Ways of Thinking* 5 ed. (London: Pearson Education, 2007).

* J. Sternin and R. Choo, "The Power of Positive Deviance," *Harvard Business Review* January-February (2000).

* J. Sternin, "Positive Deviance for Extraordinary Social and Organizational Change," in *The Change Champions Fieldguide*, ed. D. Ulrich et al. (New York: Best Practice Publications LLC, 2003), 20-37.

* S. Strogatz, *Sync: The Emerging Science of Spontaneous Order* (New York: Hyperion, 2003).

* R. Trudeau, *Introduction to Graph Theory* (New York: Dover Publications, 1993).

* A. Van de Ven and R. Garud, "The Coevolution of Technical and Institutional Events in the Development of an Innovation," in *Evolutionary Dynamics in Organizations*, ed. J. Baum and J. Singh. (New York: Oxford University Press, 1994), 425-443.

* D. Watts, *Small Worlds: The Dynamics of Networks between Order and Randomness* (Princeton: Princeton University Press, 1999).

* D. Weber and B. W. Depew, *Darwinism Evolving: System Dynamics and the Genealogy of Natural Selection* (Cambridge: MIT Press, 1994).

* B. J. West, *Fractal Physiology and Chaos in Medicine* (Singapore: World Scientific, 1990).

* B. J. West, *Where Medicine Went Wrong: Rediscovering the Path to Complexity* (Singapore: World Scientific, 2006).

* N. A. Wetzel and H. Winawer, "School-Based Community Family Therapy for Adolescents at Risk," in *Comprehensive Handbook of Psychotherapy*, ed. F. W. Kaslow, R. F. Massey, and S. D. Massey. (Philadl: John Wiley & Sons, 2002), 205-230.

- B. Zimmerman, C. Lindberg, and P. Plsek, *Edgeware: Insights from Complexity Science for Health Care Leaders* (Irving: VHA Inc., 2001).

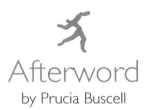

Afterword
by Prucia Buscell

Where the cliff has broken down,
Small fish gather
Under the river willow*

In nature, a verge is a place where different ecosystems come together, where abundant diversity and interaction yield a profusion of healthy living organisms. It's a place of excitement, wonder, and energetic evolutionary potential. The place where nursing and Complexity Science meet may prove to be a place that gives rise to tantalizing progress in healthcare.

Nursing is a highly complex profession where practitioners must deal with individuals and families under stress in fast-paced, technologically sophisticated environments. More than ever, it is recognized that nurses are major players in the healthcare industry. Research and analysis have shown that amount and quality of nursing care are the keys to improving patient safety and outcomes. Yet as this book emphasizes, twenty-first century nurses are required to know more and do more, and to do their jobs more quickly as compared with nurses in the twentieth century.

---

* R.H. Blyth, *Haiku, Volume 2, Spring,* Hokuseido, Japan, 1950, pp. 281.

Today's nurses also provide care in a resources-poor environment as compared to their predecessors. They must also help patients navigate a confusing world of medical treatment, care, and very complex healthcare organizations. Nurses place emphasis on the culture of safety as well as on relationships with patients, families, and colleagues. All of these areas, the editors believe, are best understood through a Complexity Science perspective.

Additional characteristics that increase the complexity of today's healthcare industry include the increasing need for interdisciplinary collaboration, opportunities for nurses to move into advanced practice and other non-traditional nursing roles, and the current nursing shortage. Technological advances have improved cure rates and extended lifespans, but have resulted in a larger number and variety of specialty providers involved in each patient's care. This can lead to a "who's on first" situation wherein no one knows who is in charge and nobody has the full picture of the patient's problems or treatments. Therefore no single person has the knowledge and ability to accurately coordinate care and communications. While nurses have always addressed this need in the past, the new Clinical Nurse Leader role was developed specifically to provide care coordination across disciplines.

As a profession, nursing is acutely aware of these challenges. There is awareness of the need for nurses to understand and apply Complexity Science principles on the part of some individuals and some professional organizations. For example, as early as 1998, in its *Essentials of Baccalaureate Education for Professional Nursing Practice*, the American Association of Colleges of Nursing (AACN) (http://www.aacn.nche.edu) recognized the forces within the healthcare industry that both increase complexity and challenge nurses' ability to provide care. The AACN has also included Complexity Science in the academic framework for Clinical Nurse Leader master's degree programs. These are indicators that the profession may be poised to embrace Complexity Science, and therefore the need for the knowledge in this book will continue to grow.

Nurses introduced to Complexity Science often report that it resonates with their experiences and that the sudden recognition of congruence in theory and real events makes them feel hopeful. According to Curt Lindberg, "Nurses who feel hopeful are more likely to engage actively in working to improve healthcare and influence policy."

Claire Lindberg notes that nurses intuitively understand Complexity Science because of who they are and what they do. People who seek nursing as a career usually want to work in environments where people have to interact to help each other. "Once they get into nursing, they find things are even more complex than they thought," she says. "When exposed to Complexity Science, they get insights into their own roles, and why things work and do not work in their environments. It gives them a structure for what they are seeing and living."

According to Sue Nash, there are additional reasons nurses need to understand Complexity Science. "People talk about a global society, and that really is what we have today. There is interconnectedness in the world, and we are just getting to the point where we can embrace it. Technology is enabling that, but there is also the recognition that we have to look to each other to help each other survive on the planet."

The scholars and practitioners who came together to produce *On the Edge: Nursing in the Age of Complexity,* represent different experiences and traditions in science, education, and healthcare. The editors of this volume hope this collection of theoretical and practical knowledge will lead nurses on a new journey of professional discovery and drive future explorations in science and healthcare. Curt Lindberg observes, "I have been struck by the genuine respect and interest complexity scientists have for nursing." He recalls that when asked why he was presenting at a nursing conference, Bruce West replied, "What nurses do is more complex than what I do as a theoretical physicist, and it is more important."

Nurses, in turn, have been impressed with West's insights into human physiology, and the potential they hold for new understandings of health and patient care. Curt Lindberg continues on to say, "My dream is that the intersection of nursing and Complexity Science will lead to improvements in both fields, and that this book will help spark a larger network of collaborators. There is real opportunity here to look at the possibilities such collaboration can generate."

A verge is the brink of progress, or the beginning of a transition to something new. It is the edge where change foments in fertile ground and evolution occurs. The principles of Complexity Science and the theory and practice of nursing together can generate creative approaches to new developments in healthcare and raise awareness of future trends. A few examples of complex challenges in the healthcare field that may benefit from a Complexity Science approach to problem solving include the rapid growth of antibiotic resistant infections, the increase in the number of people suffering from chronic illnesses, and coming changes in healthcare cost reimbursement. New emphasis on disease prevention and management, information technology, and continuing care outside of traditional institutional settings herald change as well as opportunity.

An extraordinary body of scholarship already exists on Complexity Science, so students can delve into resources with a wide array of perspectives. This book deals specifically with the confluence of nursing and complexity, and it bridges the gap between theory and the daily realities of nurses' work. This book is about giving nurses an opportunity to learn how to use insights and principles from Complexity Science to overcome current obstacles and to bring about positive change in the health and well-being of patients and families. It also addresses ways to move the profession of nursing forward. It is the editors' hope that nurses who understand Complexity Science will be both fully equipped to contribute to innovative practices and policies and to respond to new roles and new professional demands.

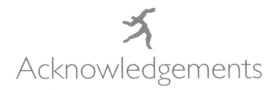

Acknowledgements

The editors of this book would like to thank the authors and contributors who gave their time and expertise to make this volume possible. We appreciate your dedication to Complexity Science and to the nursing profession!

We would also like to acknowledge two people who helped us with chapter editing, proofreading, and keeping track (well, mostly) of all documents and details involved in this editing task. To Prucia Buscell, Communications Director of Plexus Institute: Thank you for sharing your expertise in writing, editing, and Complexity Science literature among other things! To our student journalism intern from The College of New Jersey, Joseph Hannan: Thank you for joining us in this journey! Your editing and organizational skills have been tremendously helpful in keeping us on track as we pulled together the final version of the book.

Special appreciation goes to David Hutchens, who created the cover and interior design for the book. His design taste added an appealing look to some appealing content.

We'd also like to thank our families, the staff, and board members of Plexus Institute who supported and humored us through the three years it took to produce this book.

Index

A

adaptation 264
ADPIE model 215
agent-based models 264
Ruth Anderson 90, 149
appreciative inquiry 175
artificial life 264
attractor 265
    fixed point attractor 265
    periodic (limit cycle) attractor 266
    strange attractor 266
attractors 231
autopoeisis 266

B

balanced scorecard 172
basins of attraction 266
James Begun 260
bell curve 100
benard system 267
bifurcation 267
boundaries 268
Murray Bowen 188
butterfly effect 41, 268

C

caring, role in nursing 249
catastrophe theory 269
cellular automata 269
chaos 270
chaos theory 34
chunking 270
Clinical Nurse Leader 13, 14, 17, 244, 254
clinical reasoning web 222
clockware 31, 288
co-evolution 185, 190, 193, 194, 271
coherence 271
complex adaptive systems 9, 11, 30, 67, 73, 87, 131, 152, 185, 193, 197, 234, 272
complex adaptive systems, characteristics of 35
complex adaptive systems, families as an example of 190, 191
complex responsive processes 34, 41, 43, 130, 272
complexity 271

complexity science 12, 13, 14, 16, 17,
    31, 32, 50, 51, 59, 61, 62, 87, 128, 131,
    133, 135, 136, 137, 140, 143, 145, 146,
    150, 151, 173, 190, 191, 194, 196, 198,
    203, 204, 205, 206, 233, 234, 235, 242
complexity science in healthcare 9, 64,
    74
connecting activities in nursing 252
conversation circles 195
Crossing the Quality Chasm ix, 7, 29,
    164

D

deterministic system 273
difference questioning 274
dissipative structure 274
diversity 235
diversity in families 197
Doctor of Nursing Practice role 251
dynamical system 275

E

Norbert Elias 33
emergence 40, 275
equilibrium 276

F

family therapy 187, 188
family social science 187
family, definitions of 186
far-from-equilibrium 276
feedback 277
fitness landscape 277
fractal 278

G

Mary Gambino 67
game of life 269
J. Gauss 99
Murray Gell-Mann 33
genetic algorithm 278
Jeffrey Goldstein 289
graph theory 279

H

healthcare, cost of 4
HIV/AIDS 137
homeostasis and physiology 104
homeostasis, false assumptions about
    98
Cynthia Hornberger xi
human becoming theory 60
Hunterdon Medical Center 147, 150,
    154

I

industrial model of healthcare 3
information 279
initial conditions 280
instability 280
Institute of Medicine 7, 13, 29, 64, 147,
    164, 252
interaction 280

K

Stuart Kauffman 33
Kevin Kelly 270, 288
J. A. Scott Kelso i, 33
Colleen P. Kosiak vii

L

leadership competencies 241
Claire Lindberg 44
Curt Lindberg 45, 151
linear system 281
Henri Lipmanowicz 152
local interactions and quality of care 85
logical positivism 54
Edward Lorenz 33, 40, 268

M

Benoit Mandelbrot 33, 105, 106
Reuben McDaniel 87, 91
mechanistic metaphor 128
mechanistic world view and nursing 54,
    55
minimum specifications 281

N

NANDA (North American Nursing Diagnosis Association) 214
Sue Nash xiv, 206
network mapping 175
neural networks 281
Newtonian model 55, 57
Newtonian model in healthcare 28, 30, 31
San Ng 156
Florence Nightingale 58
nonlinear system 282
nonlinearity 282
novelty 282
nursing interventions classification (NIC) 214, 225
nursing outcomes classification (NOC) 214, 225
nursing shortage 138, 141

O

Outcome-Present-State Test (OPT) Model of Reflective Clinical Reasoning 216, 218, 233

P

palliative care movement 125, 136
paradox 159, 165, 167, 168
parameters 283
Vilfredo Pareto 101
partnership care delivery model 13, 18
patient safety 138, 143
Daniel Pesut 235
phase space 283
physics, history of 98
physiological time series 108
    fractals in life sciences 107
    heart rate variability (HRV) 108
    breathing rate variability (BRV) 113
    stride rate variability (SRV) 116
    Bruce West 121
Plexus Institute 147
Positive Deviance 129, 133, 138, 145, 284
postmodernism 54, 57

power laws 284
Illya Prigogine 33
primary nursing model 10

R

reductionism 30, 54, 192
redundancy 285
Linda Rusch 147, 150, 153

S

SARS 160, 169, 177
Cicely Saunders 125, 135
scale 285
scale-free network 285
scaling 107
science of unitary human beings 59
self organization 38, 74, 76, 77, 87, 152, 153, 190, 193, 194, 197, 198, 201, 231, 233, 243, 286
    self organization, example of 38
self organized criticality 286
sensitive dependence on initial conditions 287
siloed organizations 3, 4
simple, complicated and complex 26, 27, 234, 242
simulations 175
small world network 287
social networks 279
stability 288
Ralph Stacey 33, 41, 76, 130, 190, 191
storytelling 152, 221
Anthony Suchman 43
swarmware 288
symbiogenesis 288
synchronization 288
systems, family 188

T

theory of health as expanding consciousness 60
thinking - complex 229
thinking - creative 228
thinking - critical 227
thinking - systems 228, 229

time series 289
To Err is Human report 7
Total Quality Management, failure of 61
Deborah Tregunno 180
trust in nursing 247
    demand for services 246

V

variability and health 99

W

Kenneth White 260
Marjorie Wiggins 16, 20, 148
Edward O. Wilson 33

Z

Brenda Zimmerman 156, 181

2361550

Made in the USA